Dan:

Keep conquering the 🧠 ← Brain

Thank you!   Karen O.

CONTINUAL RAVING

CONTINUAL RAVING

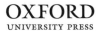

*A HISTORY OF MENINGITIS
AND THE PEOPLE WHO
CONQUERED IT*

JANET R. GILSDORF

OXFORD
UNIVERSITY PRESS

OXFORD

UNIVERSITY PRESS

Oxford University Press is a department of the University of Oxford. It furthers
the University's objective of excellence in research, scholarship, and education
by publishing worldwide. Oxford is a registered trade mark of Oxford University
Press in the UK and certain other countries.

Published in the United States of America by Oxford University Press
198 Madison Avenue, New York, NY 10016, United States of America.

Library of Congress Control Number: 2019949626
ISBN 978–0–19–067731–2

1 3 5 7 9 8 6 4 2
Printed by Sheridan Books, Inc., United States of America

To Jim for your unending patience

CONTENTS

———◆———

PREFACE

As the paint chemist Carl W. Reed observed, "You can't plan discovery." Discovery wanders, without a guide, from thought to thought and observation to observation, snaking freely in the thickets of ideas and speculations. It's the product of curiosity, the result of questions: Why? How? and What if? It can be as simple as a doctor gazing at sputum using a microscope and finding a new bacterium or as complicated as a scientist interpreting the entire genetic code of that bacterium. It's the product of hard work, serendipity, and a prepared mind built on the fruits of prior breakthroughs.

Through the ages, cadres of devoted and persistent physicians and scientists have devoted their lives to understanding the wily ways of the bacteria that cause meningitis. Theirs was the exhilarating world of discovery. This book examines their journeys—their questions, their good (and bad) fortunes, and, amid occasional moans of despair, their enthusiastic shouts of triumph.

Meningitis is a devastating disease by any measure. Before antibiotics, it resulted in death in most of the children—most victims were under 5 years old—who contracted it or led to severe neurologic damage in the very few who survived. An early step on the path to its conquest was discovery of the bacterium *Haemophilus influenzae* by the

German physician Richard Pfeiffer during the Russian influenza pandemic of 1889.

The path toward victory over meningitis continued through weedy fields populated by the mysteries of immunity and the trials and errors of new treatments. The secrets of *H. influenzae* increasingly were revealed: its susceptibility to evolving treatments, its immunology, its capsule, its DNA, and its ability to soak up new DNA and thus to create new versions of itself. While the researchers were busy researching, *H. influenzae* learned to outwit the life-saving antibiotics used to treat it. A catalogue of all of its genes was produced and, finally, the ultimate prize, a vaccine that could prevent all *H. influenzae* infections of the type b variety.

I first met both meningitis and the bacteria that cause it during my pathology and microbiology courses in medical school. They were merely abstract words to me then, a disease and a series of bacteria with tongue-twisting names: *Haemophilus influenzae, Neisseria meningitidis* (also known as meningococci), and *Streptococcus pneumoniae* (also known as pneumococci). I hadn't yet encountered them in patients. Later, during my medical school clinical training, residency in pediatrics, fellowship in pediatric infectious diseases, and the early years of my work as an infectious diseases pediatrician, I delivered medical care to many young children with meningitis and witnessed firsthand at the crib side, the terrible effects of this awful infection. Then, the *H. influenzae* type b (Hib) vaccine arrived, and because of its widespread use, Hib meningitis is now very rare in America's children. Similarly, vaccines against meningococci and pneumococci prevent many additional cases of meningitis.

As a physician and a scientist, I have great admiration for those who made the important early observations on which later findings were built. Further, *H. influenzae* and its cunning ways, its graceful beauty, its infuriating refusal to follow the rules have accompanied me throughout my professional life, and I have had the good fortune to live during the time of many of the contemporary innovations that have brought nearly complete freedom from Hib meningitis in the United States. Every one of those hard-won discoveries warranted the shouting.

ACKNOWLEDGMENTS

I am extremely grateful to the legion of scientists whose work is summarized in these pages; to the Hathitrust, without which this book wouldn't be possible; to Dan Granoff, who first taught me the beauty and wonder of *Haemophilus influenzae*; to my patients and fellow infectious diseases colleagues, who honed my understanding of the complexities of meningitis; to my readers, Jane Johnson, Danielle Lavaque-Manty, Marty Calvert, Ann Epstein, Cynthia Jalinsky, and Jim Gilsdorf, who generously offered the hard, brilliant suggestions to bring polish to this book. I deeply appreciate the efforts of Dr. Dieter Roloff, who painstakingly translated the original articles on *H. influenzae* and meningitis from German to English; and Eckart Roloff, who found the first name (Adolf) of A. Pfuhl, the German military pathologist who first described meningitis caused by *H. influenzae*.

I

Meningitis—What Is It?

TO A PEDIATRICIAN, MENINGITIS is an infection of the tissues that cover the brain and spinal cord: the dura mater, the pia mater, and the arachnoid mater. To the parents of children with this disease, it's heartbreak and terror, worry-filled days, and sleepless nights. Endless questions crowd their troubled minds: Will he survive? If she does, will she be normal? Why did this happen to my baby? Did I do something wrong?

Victims of meningitis often are healthy young children, playful, delightful kids doing typical toddler things—playing peekaboo, smearing food all over their faces, singing, dancing, giggling—until suddenly, with no explanation, they develop a fever. Their parents might give them acetaminophen and pass it off as "a virus" because viruses are so very common and kids get fevers with every little thing. By the next day, the children become cranky, satisfied with nothing. They won't eat. They refuse to play. They vomit and then become listless. All they want is to snuggle in their parents' laps, and be rocked, and feel secure. If they don't receive appropriate antibiotic treatment, things get worse quickly. The children become very sleepy and quake with seizures. Their eyes begin to move in funny directions; one eye may point at their noses while the other wanders. They then drift into a coma and don't respond to their sibling's touch, their parent's kiss, or their doctor's voice. If the meningitis is caused by bacteria, without antibiotic treatment, they almost always die.

I was a medical student when I first encountered meningitis. To me, then, it was a vague notion, a medical word without anything real

Continual Raving: A History of Meningitis and the People Who Conquered It. Janet R Gilsdorf, Oxford University Press (2020). © Oxford University Press.
DOI: 10.1093/oso/9780190677312.001.0001

connected to it, a mere term that meant an infectious process in the central nervous system. Later, as a physician-in-training in pediatrics and a young specialist in infectious diseases, I was the doctor responsible for the medical care of many, many children with meningitis. When attached to terribly ill kids, the word suddenly festered with achy, indelible meaning.

Back then, on any given day, two to three children on the pediatric ward were hooked to antibiotic drips as they underwent treatment for bacterial meningitis. Many would ultimately be released from the hospital; often, in spite of antibiotic treatment, they suffered from neurologic impairment of one type or another. The daughter of one of my resident mates had meningitis caused by the bacterium *Haemophilus influenzae*, as did the son of one of my professors. The girl suffered permanent hearing loss in one ear, and the boy had difficulty in school and failed to live up to his father's expectations. Some meningitis patients never went home at all.

When I'd examine children suffering from meningitis, I'd marvel at their peaceful appearance. Between seizures, they lay in their cribs, unmoving, unresponsive, as if asleep. Their outward calm, however, belied the vicious disease process churning inside their heads. Bacteria in the tissues surrounding their brains were replicating and spewing out their toxic factors, and the children's immune systems were battling the bacteria. Their brains swelled, the blood vessels that fed their cerebral neurons were pinched shut, and the neurons withered and then died.

In early descriptions of neurologic illnesses, seventeenth-century clinicians spoke of "phrensy," a malady characterized by fever, headache, and delirium. Most likely, patients suffering from phrensy, particularly children, had one of two different diseases. They had either meningitis, which was named first in 1828by John Abercrombie[1] and literally means inflammation of the three meningeal membranes that surround the brain, or encephalitis, which means inflammation of the brain itself, usually caused by viruses.

The venerable physician Dr. Thomas Willis poetically compared delirium to phrensy, stating, "In a *Delirium* the perturbation rais'd in the Spirits, residing in the Brain seems like undulation of Waters in a River, upon throwing in a stone; but in a *Phrensy* their commotion seems as the troublous motion of the Sea-waves raging upon a tempest" (p. 452). He went on to portray phrensy as "continual raving or a depravation of the chief faculties of the brain arising from an inflammation of the meninges with a continual fever."[2]

This description suggests that phrensy (the precursor of the modern word *frenzy*) may have referred to what we now know as seizures. Willis, a highly respected anatomist, dissected the brains of his patients who died of phrensy and found them to be inflamed, swollen, and compressed against the insides of their skulls, similar to the pathologic findings in what we now know as meningitis. He also recognized that some patients with phrensy displayed lethargy rather than raving.[3]

To Willis, the mechanisms underlying the lethargic and the manic forms of phrensy were ethereal, invoking anatomy and apparitions: "For inflamm'd Meninges, and much more swollen, greatly compress the Brain, and stop the passages of the Spirits, which causes a Lethargy; whereas in a Phrensy the Spirits are dilated above measure, the Pores of the Brain being all open'd."[2(p. 452)] We now recognize that spirits have little to do with the lethargy or seizures or any other symptoms of meningitis. Rather, these symptoms represent an alteration of central nervous system activity caused by brain swelling, which is secondary to meningeal inflammation from the infection and reduced blood flow to the nervous tissues (Figure 1.1). In short, infection → brain swelling → reduced blood flow → altered brain function → lethargy or seizures.

Early clinicians had difficulty differentiating the various types of acute brain insults: meningitis, encephalitis, brain abscess, and stroke. The Scottish physician Robert Whytt distinguished "dropsy of the brain"—fluid accumulated in the cerebral ventricles (chambers deep inside the brain) and characteristic of advanced meningitis—from other central nervous system disorders.[4] Most of the patients he described with dropsy likely had either hydrocephalus (literally water brain or water on the brain) due to congenital anatomic abnormalities that resulted in blocked cerebrospinal fluid (CSF) flow or hydrocephalus as a complication of meningitis. In patients with meningitis, unchecked inflammation from the infection interrupts the flow of the CSF that normally percolates over and through the brain as well as around the

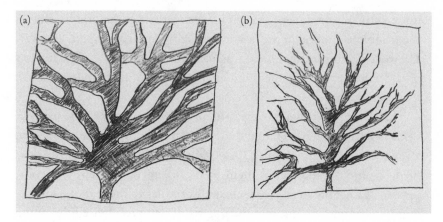

FIGURE 1.1 Cerebral edema. a. Normal brain with rich blood supply. b. Brain during meningitis with constricted blood vessels from cerebral swelling.

Drawing by the author.

spinal cord (Figure 1.2). As a result, the liquid builds up within the chambers of the cerebral ventricles and increases the pressure inside the patient's skull.

The presence of CSF), which is normally clear as spring water, around human brains was first observed during prehistoric times when trepanation [drilling holes into living people's skulls] was common practice. The purposes for this procedure are unclear, but may have involved banishing evil spirits. Many archeological skull specimens from the Neolithic Era (10,000—8000 BCE) exhibited trepans (Figure 1.3).[5]

Although the early Greek physician Hippocrates (born ca. 460 BCE) described the water surrounding the brains of children with congenital hydrocephalus[6], and the first-century Greek physician Galen of Pergamon recognized CSF as "excremental fluid" contained in the ventricles of the brain[7], this knowledge was lost in the shadows of history until 1764, when the Italian physician Domenico Cotugno described the space between the dura mater and the spinal cord as being filled "not by a thick vapor; but with water like that which the pericardium contains about the heart; or such as fills the hollows of the ventricles of

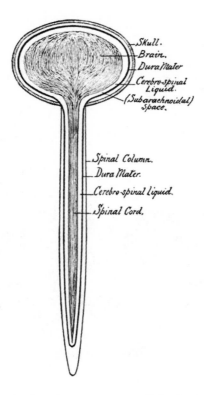

Skull.
Brain.
Dura Mater
Cerebro-spinal Liquid.
(Subarachnoidal) Space.

Spinal Column.
Dura Mater.
Cerebro-spinal Liquid.
Spinal Cord.

FIGURE 1.2 Schematic showing structures of the brain and spinal cord, including the meninges.

From Howell WH. *A Text-Book of Physiology, for Medical Students and Physicians.* Philadelphia: Saunders; 1905:554.

the brain, the labyrinth of the ear, or other cavities of the body, which are impervious to the air." —[8(p. 355)]

By the early 1800s, excessive buildup of CSF, as occurs in hydrocephalus, was recognized as a pathologic state and thought to complicate many illnesses. Thus, evacuation of the fluid was often recommended as a cure for hydrocephalus and was based on treatments for unrelated conditions that involved the removal of fluid from other organs.[4] Early efforts to evacuate CSF were awkward, invasive, and dangerous. They included direct evacuation by skull trepanation as well as a number of indirect techniques, such as purging with jalop (a Mexican purgative plant), rhubarb, calomel (mercury chloride), or scammony (bindweed), as well as bloodletting, diuretics, leeches, mineral acids mixed

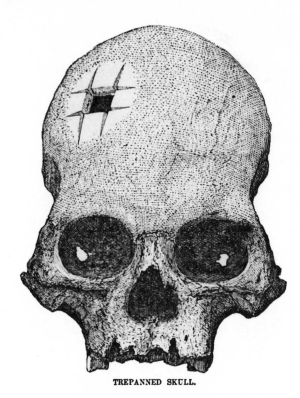

TREPANNED SKULL.

FIGURE 1.3 Trepanned skull found in 1871 in a cemetery in Peru.
From Squier EG. *Peru; Incidents of Travel and Exploration in the Land of the Incas.*
London: Macmillan; 1877:457.

with squill (a plant of the lily family), or digitalis.[9] Most importantly, such treatments would have been completely ineffective.

Although physicians could readily obtain CSF during examinations of brains after death, obtaining premortem fluid for diagnosis of a patient's medical problem was difficult. Finally, in 1891, the physician Heinrich Quincke performed the first spinal tap on a 21-month-old boy with meningitis; Quincke used a technique similar to that still practiced today.[10] After he inserted a cannula through the skin of the boy's lower back and into the space between the third and fourth lumbar vertebral bones to a depth of 2 cm, a few milliliters of watery fluid dripped from the needle's hub (Figure 1.4). Quincke subsequently performed the procedure on other patients with purulent meningitis and described the

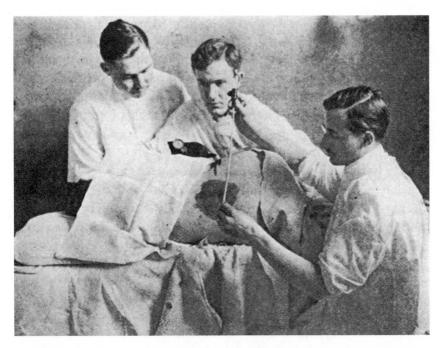

FIGURE 1.4 Performing a lumbar puncture. The patient is lying on his side with his knees curled toward his chest and his bowed head on the left. The skin of his back has been swabbed with a dark-colored antiseptic liquid (iodine), and the physicians have inserted a needle through the skin, between the vertebrae (bones of the spinal column) and then into the spinal canal. The pressure in the canal is being measured with the long tube.

From Sophian A. *Epidemic Cerebrospinal Meningitis.* St. Louis, MO: Mosby; 1913:171.

classic characteristics of infected spinal fluid: high protein, low glucose, and pleocytosis (elevated numbers of white blood cells).[11,12]

Before that first spinal tap, the diagnosis of meningitis was based on clinical signs and symptoms (fever, lethargy, stiff neck, seizures) and could be confirmed only by pathologic examination of the brains of deceased patients during an autopsy. Since the advent of the spinal tap, the diagnosis of meningitis rests on examination of the CSF for evidence of inflammation, as indicated by (1) increased white blood cells, primarily polymorphonuclear cells (normal 0–5/mm^3); (2) decreased glucose level (normal > 70 mg/100 mL), thought to be from decreased transport of glucose from the blood to the fluid and from utilization of glucose in the fluid by the white cells and bacteria; (3) increased protein level (normal < 50 mg/100 mL) from proteins seeping out of the blood into the spinal fluid and from decomposing cells and bacteria; and (4) the presence of the microbes that cause the infection by growing them in bacteriologic culture or observing them on Gram stain through a microscope. Even today, analysis of CSF for chemical, cellular, and bacteriologic abnormalities remains the *only* definitive way to diagnose bacterial meningitis; sophisticated radiographic studies such as magnetic resonance imaging (MRI) or computed tomography (CT) scans provide very detailed images of the brain structures but cannot define with certainty the cause of an inflammatory process or the microorganism causing an infection.

A variety of microbes, such as fungi, viruses, or bacteria, or noninfectious, inflammatory processes may cause meningitis.[13] Fungal meningitis is rarely seen in healthy individuals but may occur in patients who are immunosuppressed; in those with metal or plastic devices inserted into their central nervous systems; or in those inadvertently injected with medication contaminated with mold.[14] Meningitis caused by viruses is common and, with a few exceptions, doesn't require antimicrobial treatment. Viral meningitis is for the most part benign and spontaneously resolves without permanent neurologic complications.

Many different types of bacteria can cause meningitis in children, including *Mycobacterium tuberculosis*, which was a leading cause of meningitis in the United States before tuberculosis was fairly well controlled during the early to mid-twentieth century. It remains, however, a significant cause of meningitis in resource-limited countries. More recently, among healthy but unimmunized young children, the most common causes are three species of bacteria: *Neisseria meningitidis* (meningococci); *Streptococcus pneumoniae* (pneumococci); and *Haemophilus influenzae*, abbreviated *H. influenzae*, and earlier called *Bacillus influenzae*, abbreviated *B. influenzae*. All three of these bacteria normally live, without causing infections, in the nose and throat of healthy children and adults (i.e. carriers). In carrier children who are not immunized, any of these three bacteria may wander from the respiratory mucosa into their bloodstream, and the blood then ferries the bacteria to the capillary beds of many tissues, including, occasionally, the meninges. Thus, bacterial meningitis begins.

The first cases of bacterial meningitis were described during outbreaks of the disease in the early 1800s. Between January and April 1805, Gaspard Vieusseux, a physician from near Geneva, Switzerland, documented 33 fatal cases of patients with weakness, feeble pulse, vomiting, and convulsions. In those who died within 24 hours of getting sick, purple patches quickly covered their skin, signifying subcutaneous bleeding. An unknown number of additional patients had the infection but survived, as the course of the disease was said to be "very rapid [with] termination by death or cure."[3(p. 421)15]

During an outbreak of meningitis the next year in New Bedford, Massachusetts, the doctors Lothario Danielson and Elias Mann reported dramatic, livid purple patches on the skin of nine children with fever, vomiting, and rapid progression to coma.[16,17] In an additional report of this outbreak, the purple rash was described in great detail by the medical student Nathan Strong:

> Blind haemorrhages, or those where the blood flowing from the vessels of the skin, is detained beneath the cuticle, forming petechial [purple] spots. ... So frequent indeed was this species of haemorrhage during the first season in which the disease prevailed, that it was considered as one of its most striking characteristicks [sic].[18(p. 10)]

The characteristic rash gave rise to the name petechial or spotted fever. Although these early reports could not identify the cause of the infections, the presence of purple skin patches (known today as purpura) as well as the clustering of those early cases in time and place suggest that *Neisseria meningitidis* (meningococci) was the cause.

Because these cases of purple rashes and meningitis tended to occur over a short period of time in neighborhoods and communities, the disease was also called "epidemic meningitis." The bacterial cause of epidemic meningitis was finally discovered in 1884 when the Italian physicians Marchiafava and Celli observed small round (cocci) bacteria (characteristic of meningococci) inside the white blood cells of a spinal fluid specimen,[19] strongly suggesting that the patient's meningitis was caused by meningococci. Three years later, Dr. Anton Weichselbaum grew on agar plates bacteria from CSF samples of six patients with epidemic meningitis; he described the germs as gram-*negative* (stained pink) cocci, distinguishable from the gram-*positive* (stained purple) cocci (pneumococci) that were known to cause pneumonia. Thus meningococci were clearly established as the cause of epidemic meningitis.[20]

Meningitis caused by *H. influenzae* was first described by Dr. Adolf Pfuhl, a German military pathologist, several months after Dr. Richard Pfeiffer reported finding that organism, which he called "influenza bacilli" in the bronchi of patients with Russian influenza.[21,22] Pneumococci were first identified in patients with meningitis 6 years later, in 1898.[23]

Although physicians continued to observe bacteria consistent with *H. influenzae*, or Pfeiffer's bacilli, in the brains of children who died of apparent Russian influenza,[22,24] merely *seeing* structures that look like bacilli under the microscope, instead of *culturing* them on agar, left their exact identification in doubt. Finally, S. Slawyk, a military physician in Berlin, succeeded in growing Pfeiffer's influenza bacilli in pure culture—no other kinds of bacteria grew—from the CSF as well as from the blood of a 9-month-old boy with meningitis. At autopsy, the same bacilli were cultured from the left ventricle of the boy's brain as well as from his lungs and an ankle abscess, indicating widespread bacterial infection.[25] To counter skeptical colleagues who questioned the identification of the bacteria, the microbes from Slawyk's patient were verified as influenza bacilli by Pfeiffer himself.[26]

By 1911, a growing number of cases of meningitis from which Pfeiffer's influenza bacilli, also called *Bacillus influenzae*, had grown from the CSF were published in the medical literature.[25–28] Whether these meningitis cases were actually caused by influenza bacilli is difficult to know because several occurred in adults (most patients with true *H. influenzae* meningitis are young children), and several had multiple bacterial pathogens isolated on bacterial culture.

It was the carefully detailed studies of Dr. Martha Wollstein that confirmed Pfeiffer's bacillus as an important cause of meningitis.[29] During the course of 1 year, Wollstein saw slender, rod-shaped bacteria in the spinal fluid specimens of eight children with meningitis at Babies'

Hospital in New York. She described the spinal fluid of each child as turbid or very turbid (rather than its normal crystal clear appearance), and in patients with repeated spinal taps during their illnesses, the fluid became more turbid over time. On the last day of one child's life, the spinal fluid consisted of thick pus. Wollstein grew Pfeiffer's bacillus, *B. influenzae*, in pure culture from blood or spinal fluid of each of the eight children she reported.

Eleven years later, in 1922, Dr. Thomas Rivers compiled the most comprehensive series of "influenzal meningitis" patients reported to date.[30] Besides describing 23 children with "influenzal meningitis" admitted to the Harriet Lane Home in Baltimore, Maryland, from 1913 to 1921, Rivers reviewed all 220 influenzal meningitis cases described in the medical literature and observed that, amazingly, a few survived. The mortality rate, however, was very high, at 92%. The first reported child who recovered from influenzal meningitis was a 9-year-old boy with at least 8 days of somnolence and severe headache and 3 days of stiff neck who, following a spinal tap, became afebrile. Several days later he was both demanding toys and reading a picture book. He was discharged from the hospital as cured.[31] Of the 17 patients reported as recovered in Rivers's paper, twelve were over age 2 years, and four demonstrated neurologic damage that included facial paralysis, hemiplegia, blindness, or deafness.

In addition to describing survivors, Rivers provided the first comprehensive description of the symptoms and clinical courses of patients with *B. influenzae* meningitis. He noted that the diagnosis was difficult to make on clinical grounds alone, and the disease was indistinguishable from "epidemic meningitis" (caused by meningococci), particularly since the characteristic purple rash of epidemic meningitis could occasionally be seen in patients with influenzal meningitis. Further, influenzal meningitis also mimicked tuberculous meningitis; increased intracranial pressure seen in both infections could result in paralysis of the eye muscles, irregular respirations, and extreme bulging of the fontanel (the "soft spot" at the top of an infant's head). In patients with influenzal meningitis, the body temperature was elevated either continuously or intermittently, and febrile periods could alternate with periods of normal temperature.

The following is from Rivers's 1922 article[30(p. 111)]:

Case 5.—H. M., white female, 7 months old, became drowsy and feverish three weeks before admission to the hospital. At first there was a slight discharge from the nose. The family physician treated the baby for bronchitis in spite of the fact that she had no signs of it, not even a cough until a few days before coming to the hospital. One week before admission projectile vomiting after each feeding developed and three days before admission the head became retracted [tipped back]. The patient was admitted Jan. 21, 1919. The physical examination showed a conscious, hyperesthetic [irritable] baby with a stiff neck and a retracted head, no discharge from the nose or ears, anisocoria [unequal size of the pupils], indefinite signs of pneumonia in right interscapular [between the scapula bones] region, exaggerated deep reflexes. White blood cell count was 50,880 [highly elevated]. The spinal fluid was very thick and purulent. Gram-negative bacilli were seen in the smears. Culturally, these were influenza bacilli. The blood culture remained sterile. The child gradually became worse and began to have numerous convulsions before she died January 26. A necropsy was not allowed.

Such was a typical story of a baby with meningitis: young child; developed fever and drowsiness, vomiting and stiff neck; had a spinal tap that revealed too many white blood cells (evidence of inflammation of the meninges) and grew influenzal bacilli on spinal fluid culture. In the end, most children, including Rivers's patient in Case 5, developed convulsions and died (Figures 1.5 and 1.6).

Thomas Rivers was born into a farming family in Jonesboro, Georgia, in 1888.[32] He was introduced to medicine early, as he developed typhoid fever when he was 12 years old and was confined to his bed for 4 months. He survived in spite of, rather than because of, the popular treatments of the day: starvation and ice-water baths.[33]

After Tom graduated summa cum laude from Emory College, his father requested his return to Jonesboro to assist with the family businesses. Tom chose, instead, to go to medical school. During his second year in medicine at Johns Hopkins University, he noticed that his left

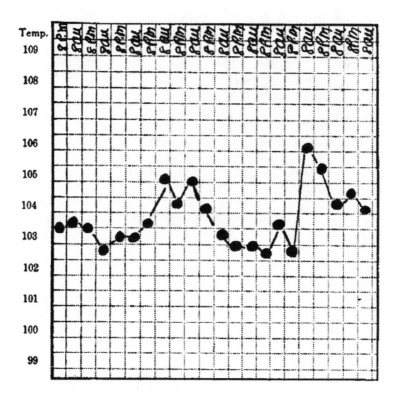

FIGURE 1.5 Fever curve from Rivers's Case 5 patient with influenzal meningitis.

From Rivers TM. Influenzal Meningitis. *American Journal of Diseases of Children.* 1922;24:102–124.

hand was weak, and its muscles showed signs of atrophy. He was given the diagnosis of Aran-Duchenne muscular atrophy and told that the disease would run a rapidly fatal course. Tom dropped out of medical school and returned to Jonesboro. As he wrote, "After mooning around for a while, I kind of got fed up waiting to die."[33(p. 11)] He subsequently spent 18 months in Panama as a laboratory assistant and then returned to medical school at Hopkins, graduating in 1915. His hand remained weak, but it didn't interfere with his work in any way. Since it didn't progress and he didn't die, he had obviously received an incorrect diagnosis.

When Rivers graduated from medical school, pediatrics was not a well-respected field of medicine, and the medical care of children was

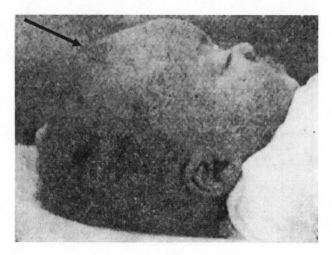

FIGURE 1.6 Bulging fontanelle (arrow) from Rivers's Case 5 patient with influenzal meningitis.

From Rivers TM. Influenzal Meningitis. *American Journal of Diseases of Children.* 1922;24:102–124.

not highly regarded in clinical circles. Its practitioners were dismissed as "baby feeders." Nevertheless, Tom chose a career in children's medicine because "adults have a way of lying to their doctors. ... Children, on the other hand, have a way of always telling the truth. ... They do just what comes handy, whether it's eating or peeing on the floor. I liked pediatrics because children appealed to me. I couldn't stand neurotic women and lying men."[33(p. 38)]

In Rivers's early experience in pediatrics, all children with meningitis died. During a dispute about how to deal with a patient with meningitis, Dr. John Howland, the chief pediatrician at Hopkins, insisted Rivers, a young intern, refrain from telling the parents of his patient that their child would die. (Figure 1.7). " 'As soon as you do,' Howland had said, 'it [the baby!] will get well and they will hold it against you.' Bless my soul, if this kid with influenzal meningitis didn't get well. He was the only case I saw that ever lived. I will admit that he was deaf for the rest of his life, but he did live, and I learned my lesson.' "[33(p. 49)]

Rivers's pediatric training in Baltimore was interrupted by World War I, and he completed his military service at Fort Sam Houston, studying

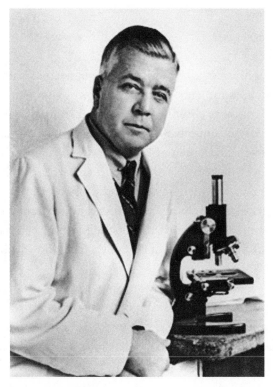

FIGURE 1.7 Dr. Thomas Rivers.

Source: US Government: https://commons.wikimedia.org/wiki/File:Thomas_Milton_Rivers.png.

outbreaks of measles and pneumonia.[34] This experience awakened his muse for research. After the war he joined the staff of the Rockefeller Institute in New York, where he built a highly successful career in the emerging field of virology. In 1926, Rivers was asked to review the status of viruses in a talk to the Society of American Bacteriologists. He began the talk by saying, "In all fields of work, times come when one must stop and take thought. New facts, new ideas, and new suggestions alter lines of endeavor in every field of research." [35(p. 217)] He stated that viral infections could be inferred because they could be transferred from one animal to another but could not be cultured on laboratory media. Then he went on to unequivocally summarize the new understanding of how viruses live: "Viruses appear to be obligate parasites in the sense that their reproduction is dependent on living cells."[35(p. 228)] Thus, a new day in infectious diseases had dawned. In 1937, Rivers revisited the causation of bacterial diseases to consider its differences from the causation of viral diseases.[36]

Although he was described as irascible, pugnacious, and stubbornly inflexible during arguments,[37] Tom Rivers was also a fun-loving guy. His right eardrum was chronically perforated from childhood, and he claimed to have won a number of bets by literally blowing smoke out of that ear.[33] He was also a man of high integrity. When he found a mistake in a paper he had published, he told a colleague that he was going to retract the paper, which would be an honorable, but unpleasant, move for a scientist. The colleague suggested he *not* retract the paper, as it "would take fifteen years for anyone else to find out" that the information was wrong. Rivers said of his colleague, "I don't think Noguchi was honest."[38(p. 441)]

In his later years, Rivers served as the medical director of the National Foundation for Infantile Paralysis (polio) and was its vice president for medical affairs until his death from lung cancer in 1962 at age 73. He and his wife of 40 years, Theresa Riefele, had no children. Rivers is buried in Arlington National Cemetery.[32]

Before the advent of antibiotics, meningitis was a dreadful infection by any standard; many of its victims were young children, and almost all died, succumbing to the disease from days to 6 weeks, or sometimes longer, after the onset of their illness. Incredibly, patients occasionally survived but were often left with varying degrees of neurologic damage.

In the winter of 1882, when she was 19 months old, the writer, lecturer, and political activist Helen Keller (Figures 1.8, 1.9, 1.10) suffered a devastating illness. In her words, from her autobiography: "In the dreary month of February came the illness which closed my eyes and ears and plunged me into the unconsciousness of a new-born baby." Her illness was said by her doctors to be "congestion of the stomach and brain."[39(p. 7)]

The disease that left Helen deaf and blind, and yet intellectually intact, was consistent with what was then known as "brain fever," a term commonly used in nineteenth-century literature. It had emerged as a replacement for the word *phrensy* and referred to inflammation of the

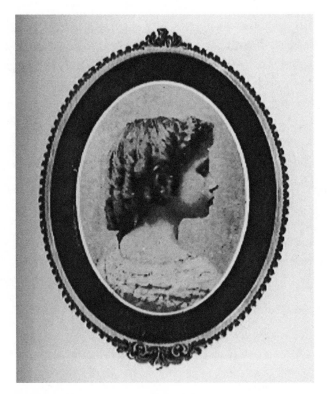

FIGURE 1.8 Helen Keller, age 7 years.

From *The Story of My Life,* edited by JA Macy. New York: Doubleday, Page; 1905:22.

brain.[40] The symptoms were described as "a vehement pyrexia [fever], a violent, deep-seated headache, a redness turgescence [swelling] of the face and eyes, an impatience of light or noise, a constant watching, and a delirium impetuous and furious."[41(p. 218)]

Brain fever was thought to always be associated with "marked inflammations of membranous parts" [41(p. 294)] of the brain, and the nomenclature is consistent with the common use of the word *fever* at that time, often meaning a form of disease, such as typhoid fever, yellow fever, scarlet fever, rheumatic fever, or breakbone fever, rather than an elevated body temperature.

Many citations that discuss Helen Keller's illness declared, without attribution, that historians and physicians believed she had scarlet fever or meningitis or less likely diagnoses such as typhoid fever, rubella, or encephalitis.[42] Scarlet fever, which has been readily recognized by

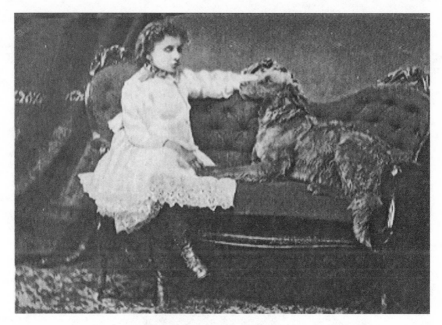

FIGURE 1.9 Helen Keller and her dog, Jumbo.
In *The Story of My Life*, edited by JA Macy. New York: Doubleday, Page; 1905:32.

physicians since the seventeenth century, always presents with fever, sore throat, and a prominent rash; at the end of the infection, the skin often peels, similar to a snake shedding its skin.[43] Waves of this illness swept through the United States from 1840 to 1877, with high mortality rates, but by 1882, the year of Helen Keller's illness, both cases and deaths were in decline.[44]

In her book, Helen Keller states that during her illness, "I ... turned my eyes, so dry and hot, to the wall, away from the once-loved light."[39(p. 7)] Such light sensitivity was a characteristic of meningitis as clearly described a century earlier in patients with "dropsy of the brain."[4] When her doctors spoke of "congestion of the stomach," they may have referred to vomiting, a common symptom of meningitis. And by "congestion of the brain," her doctors may have speculated, based on what they knew from patients who died of meningitis, that she had "congestion" of the fluid in her cerebral ventricles secondary to inflammation of the meninges. At that time, congestion of the brain would have been a pathologic observation only made at autopsy.

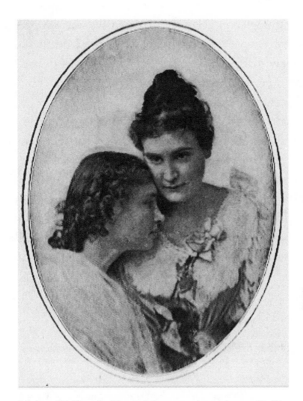

FIGURE 1.10 Helen Keller (left) and her teacher, Anne Sullivan.
Photograph by Falk, 1895. From *The Story of My Life*, edited by JA Macy.
New York: Doubleday, Page; 1905: frontispiece.

If Keller had meningitis, which bacteria would have caused it? Before antibiotic treatment became available, meningitis caused by pneumococci was uniformly fatal.[27,28] The mortality rates from *H. influenzae* meningitis were very high (97%) and from meningococcal meningitis moderately high (60%–80%).[45] Among survivors of both influenzal, as Rivers noted, and meningococcal meningitis, a few patients with deafness or blindness were reported.[30,46]

Could Helen Keller have had both meningitis and scarlet fever? Scarlet fever is occasionally, but rarely, associated with the development of meningitis and is usually the result of spread of group A streptococci (the bacteria that cause scarlet fever) to the meninges from an infected middle ear. Reports in the 1930s of over 17,000 cases of scarlet fever recorded only 19 cases of meningitis, and one of these patients recovered, with no neurologic sequelae.[47] An extensive review of scarlet fever in 1904 revealed no evidence of partial or total deafness as sequelae, and the review made no mention of blindness.[43] On the other hand, streptococci were reported as the cause of less than 1%,[28] 4%,[27] and 7%[48] of all meningitis cases.

Indeed, considering Helen Keller's young age at the time of her illness, her symptoms of prolonged fever and light sensitivity, and her specific neurologic sequelae (complete visual and hearing loss), she likely had bacterial meningitis. Scarlet fever itself isn't associated with deaf-blindness and would have easily been diagnosed by her physician. Thus, the evidence suggests she suffered from meningococcal or, possibly, *H. influenzae* meningitis (or, less likely, group A streptococcal meningitis) and was one of the fortunate, rare, survivors.

References

1. Abercrombie J. *Pathological and Practical Researches on Diseases of the Brain and the Spinal Cord.* Edinburgh: Waugh and Innes; 1828.
2. Willis T. *London Practice of Physick or the Whole Practical Part of Physick Contained in the Works of Dr. Willis.* London: Baffet and Crook; 1685.
3. Tyler KL. A History of Bacterial Meningitis. In: Aminoff MJ, Boller F, Swaab DF, eds. *Handbook of Clinical Neurology* (Vol. 95). Amsterdam: Elsevier; 2009:417–433.
4. Whytt R. *Observations on the Dropsy in the Brain.* Edinburgh: Balfour, Auld, and Smellie; 1768.
5. Alt KW, Jeunesse C, Buitrago-Tellez CH, Wachter R, Boes E, Pichler SL. Evidence for Stone Age Cranial Surgery. *Nature.* 1997;387(6631):360.
6. Hippocrates. *The Genuine Works of Hippocrates* (Vols. 1 and 2). Translated by F Adams. New York: Wood; 1886.
7. Hajdu SI. Opera Omnia as Cited in A Note from History: Discovery of Cerebrospinal Fluid. *Annals of Clinical Laboratory Science.* 2003;33(3):334–336.
8. Di Ieva A, Yasargil MG. Liquor Cotunnii: The History of Cerebrospinal Fluid in Domenico Cotugno's Work. *Neurosurgery.* 2008;63(2):352–358.
9. Shearman W. *An Essay on the Nature, Causes, and Treatment of Water in the Brain.* London: Underwood; 1825.
10. Quincke HI. Die Lumbalpunction des Hydrocephalus. *Berliner klinische Wochenschrift.* 1891;28(September 28):929–933, 965–968.
11. Uiterwijk A, Koehler PJ. A History of Acute Bacterial Meningitis. *Journal of the History of the Neurosciences.* 2012;21(3):293–313.

12. Wilkins RH. Neurosurgical Classics—XXXI. *Journal of Neurosurgery.* 1965;22(3):294–308.

13. van de Beek D, de Gans J, Tunkel AR, Wijdicks EFM. Community-Acquired Bacterial Meningitis in Adults. *New England Journal of Medicine.* 2006;354(1):44–53.

14. Kainer MA, Reagan DR, Nguyen DB, et al. Fungal Infections Associated with Contaminated Methylprednisolone in Tennessee. *New England Journal of Medicine.* 2012;367(23):2194–2203.

15. Vieusseux M. Mémoire su la Maladie qui a Regné a Genêve au Printemps de 1804. *Journal de Médecine, Chirurgie, Pharmacie.* 1805;11:163.

16. Danielson L, Mann E. The History of a Singular and Very Mortal Disease. In: *Medical and Agricultural Registrar* (Vol. 1). Boston: Manning and Loring; 1806:5.

17. Danielson L, Mann E. The First American Account of Cerebrospinal Meningitis. *Reviews of Infectious Diseases.* 1983;5(5):969–972.

18. Strong N. *An Inaugural Dissertation on the Disease Termed Petechial, or Spotted Fever.* Hartford, CT: Gleason; 1810.

19. Marchiafava E, Celli. A. Spra i Micrococchi Della Meningite Cerebrospinale Epidemica. *Gazz degli Ospedali.* 1884;5:59.

20. Weichselbaum A. Ueber die Aetiologie der Akuten Meningitis Cerebrospinalis *Fortschritte der Medizin.* 1887;5:573–583.

21. Pfuhl A. VI. Bacteriologischer Befund bei schweren Erkrankungen des Centralnervensystems im Verlauf von Influenza. *Berliner klinische Wochenschrift.* 1892;39(September 26):979–983.

22. Pfuhl A. VII. Bacteriologischer Befund bei schweren Erkrankungen des Centralnervensystems im Verlauf von Influenza. *Berliner klinische Wochenschrift.* 1892;40(October 3):1009–1011.

23. Fraenkel E. Beitrag zur Lehre von den Erkrankungen des Centralnervensystems bei Acuten Infectionsfrankheiten. *Zeitschrift für Hygiene und Infektionskrankheiten.* 1898;27:315–346.

24. Nauwerck. Influenza und Encephalitis. *Deutche Medizinische Wochenschrift.* 1895;21(June 20):393–397.

25. Slawyk S. Ein Fall von Allgemeininfection mit Influenzabacillen. *Zeitschrift für Hygiene und Infektionskrankheiten.* 1899;21:443–448.

26. Adams SS. Grip Meningitis. *Archives of Pediatrics.* 1907;24(10):721–732.

27. Dunn CH. Cerebrospinal Meningitis, Its Etiology, Diagnosis, Prognosis and Treatment. *American Journal of Diseases of Children.* 1911;1(2):95–112.

28. Holt LE. Observations on Three Hundred Cases of Acute Meningitis in Infants and Young Children. *American Journal of Diseases of Children.* 1911;1(1):26–36.

29. Wollstein M. Influenzal Meningitis and Its Experimental Production. *American Journal of Diseases of Children.* 1911;1(1):42–58.

30. Rivers TM. Influenzal Meningitis. *American Journal of Diseases of Children.* 1922;24(2):102–124.

31. Langer J. Meningitis Cerebrospinalis Suppurative, bedingt durch Influenzabacillin. *Jahrbuch für Kinderheilkunde.* 1901;53:91–98.

32. Horsfall FL. *Thomas Milton Rivers.* Washington, DC: National Academy of Sciences; 1965.

33. Benison S. *Tom Rivers: Reflections on a Life in Medicine and Science.* Cambridge, MA: MIT Press; 1967.

34. American Philosophical Society. *Thomas M. Rivers Papers.* 1971. http://www. amphilsoc.org/collections/view?docId=ead/Mss.B.R52-ead.xml;query=rivers; brand=default. Accessed October 20, 2016.

35. Rivers TM. Filterable Viruses: A Critical Review. *Journal of Bacteriology.* 1927;14(4):217–258.

36. Rivers TM. Viruses and Koch's Postulates. *Journal of Bacteriology.* 1937;33(1):1–12.

37. Shope RE. Thomas Milton Rivers 1888–1962. *Journal of Bacteriology.* 1962;84(3):385–388.

38. Barry JM. *The Great Influenza: The Epic Story of the Deadliest Plague in History.* New York: Viking; 2004.

39. Keller HA. *The Story of My Life.* New York: Doubleday, Page; 1902.

40. Peterson AC. Brain Fever in Nineteenth-Century Literature: Fact and Fiction. *Victorian Studies.* 1976;19(4):445–464.

41. Cullen W. *First Lines of the Practice of Physic* (Vol. 1, 3rd ed.). Edinburgh: Creech; 1781.

42. Gilsdorf JR. Into Darkness and Silence: What Caused Helen Keller's Deafblindness? *Clinical Infectious Diseases.* 2018;67(9):1445–1449.

43. Corlett WT. *A Treatise on the Acute, Infectious Exanthemata: Including Variola, Rubeola, Scarlatina, Rubella, Varicella, and Vaccinia, with Especial Reference to Diagnosis and Treatment.* Philadelphia: Davis; 1904.

44. Katz AR, Morens DM. Severe Streptococcal Infections in Historical Perspective. *Clinical Infectious Diseases.* 1992;14(1):298–307.

45. Flexner S, Jobling JW. An Analysis of Four Hundred Cases of Epidemic Meningitis Treated with the Anti-Meningitis Serum. *The Journal of Experimental Medicine.* 1908;10(5):690–733.

46. Beeson PB, Westerman E. Cerebrospinal Fever and Sulphonamides. *British Medical Journal.* 1943;1(4294):497.

47. Gordon JE, Top FH. Streptococcus Meningitis in Scarlet Fever. *The Journal of Pediatrics.* 1935;6(6):770–783.

48. Neal JB. Influenzal Meningitis. *Archives of Pediatrics.* 1921 38(1):1–10.

2

The Flu and Richard Pfeiffer

TO APPRECIATE THE SCIENTIFIC discoveries that ultimately conquered meningitis, we must return to the autumn of discontent, when 1889 was about to become 1890: The Russian influenza raged across Earth. Its victims were healthy one day and wracked with fevers of 104°F the next. They suffered screaming headaches and coughed until they vomited. Their throats were raw, their eyes hurt, and their muscles ached as if they'd been run over by a wagon filled with rocks. They had shaking chills. They couldn't eat. If they were very young or very old or in otherwise poor health, sometimes they died. Occasionally, in spite of being fit and well, they died anyway. It was called a "pandemic," implying that the disease was worldwide, lasted a long time, and was terrible. Indeed, the Russian influenza pandemic was all those things, and no one at that time, not physicians, not scientists, knew what caused it.

The term *influenza* comes from the Italian word *influenza*, which literally means "influence of the stars in the heavens." The name arose in the 1700s because that disease was thought to arise from astral forces. In earlier times, it was called epidemic catarrh (runny nose) and, in French, grippe (sometimes anglicized to grip). Influenza was first mentioned in the English language to describe an illness in 1743 that afflicted many citizens of Rome.[1] Sporadic cases couldn't be distinguished from what we now call colds, so the name was generally applied to respiratory illnesses that occurred among large numbers of people during epidemics. No matter what it was called, the Russian flu was miserable for those who contracted it.

Continual Raving: A History of Meningitis and the People Who Conquered It. Janet R Gilsdorf, Oxford University Press (2020). © Oxford University Press. DOI: 10.1093/oso/9780190677312.001.0001

Influenza outbreaks have been recorded since the twelfth century, and major pandemics were documented in 1803, 1833, 1837–1838, and 1847–1848.[2] The world, however, had been free of widespread influenza for nearly four decades when the Russian pandemic descended on it during the spring of 1889 (Figure 2.1). Despite its name, the Russian flu was first recognized in three widely disparate locales: Turkestan, Athabasca (northern Canada), and Greenland. Then in the early fall, it arrived in St. Petersburg, a thriving port city and railway hub from which it sped around the globe in only 4 months, and it didn't stop. Rather than extinguishing by spring of the next year, as happens with most flu epidemics, it popped up for several additional years, with waves in the winters of 1890 to 1894.[3] Although the influenza was bad during that pandemic, the weather was surprisingly good,[2] which ran counter to the then-prevailing myths that meteorological conditions or

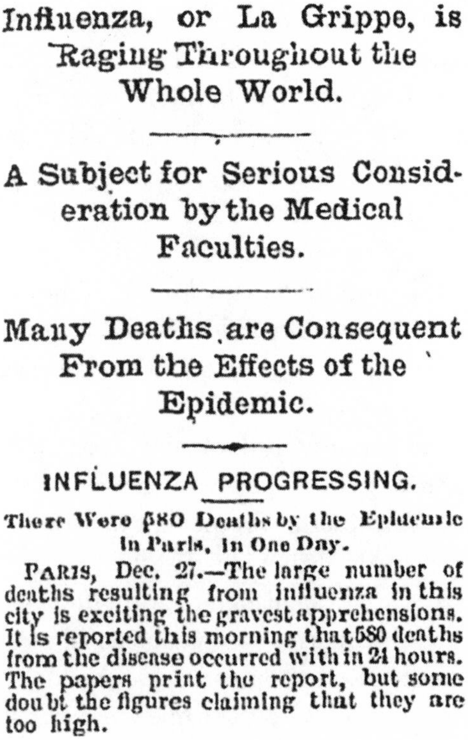

Influenza, or La Grippe, is Raging Throughout the Whole World.

A Subject for Serious Consideration by the Medical Faculties.

Many Deaths are Consequent From the Effects of the Epidemic.

INFLUENZA PROGRESSING.

There Were 580 Deaths by the Epidemic in Paris, in One Day.

PARIS, Dec. 27.—The large number of deaths resulting from influenza in this city is exciting the gravest apprehensions. It is reported this morning that 580 deaths from the disease occurred within in 24 hours. The papers print the report, but some doubt the figures claiming that they are too high.

FIGURE 2.1 World news of the Russian influenza pandemic.

From In the World. *The Gazette Democrat* (Leadville, CO), December 1889.

natural disasters, such as cold winds, winter haze, or spewing volcanos, caused influenza.

No one was too rich, too noble, or too important to escape the Russian flu. Amadeo I, the duke of Aosta, of Savoy (Italy), perished from it, as did Empress Augusta of Germany and the German priest and theologian Johann Ignaz von Döllinger. Five-year-old King Alfonso of Spain nearly died, while Czar Alexander III of Russia was said to have it twice, and the prime minister of the United Kingdom, Lord Salisbury, was incapacitated for weeks.[4] Toward the other end of the social spectrum, in Great Britain influenza attacked officers of the London post office, the staff of the Bank of England, students and workers at the Schools for Imbecile Children at Darenth, inmates at the Wormwood Scrubs and the Birmingham Prisons, patients at the Winson Green Lunatic Asylum, and detainees at the Kerrison Reformatory in Suffolk.[2]

In 1890, during the peak of the Russian flu in London, fatalities were high, estimated at 6,638 deaths per million people (Figure 2.2),

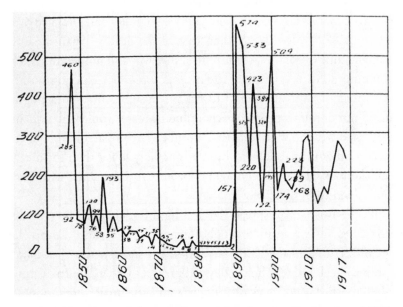

FIGURE 2.2 Death rates from influenza by date in England and Wales. The 1890–1893 peak represents the Russian flu.

From Vaughan WT. *Influenza, an Epidemiologic Study.* Baltimore: American Journal of Hygiene; 1921:48ff.

and doctors and nurses were among the most often afflicted.[2] Although relatively few British were hospitalized, they clamored to outpatient clinics for the treatment of the day, which consisted mainly of sali-cylate of soda (essentially aspirin) and strychnine.[3] Postal delivery was curtailed for weeks, and railway and telegraph services were disrupted. Infected employees worried about losing their jobs, and their inclin-ation to continue working while ill likely contributed to the spread of the disease. Less dramatically, but no less important, many of the English patients, on convalescence, were depressed, in debt, and incap-able of performing their everyday tasks. This was particularly true for the "work girls" (meaning unknown), who, according to the January 25, 1890, *Daily News*, were left "pale, listless, and full of fear"[3(p. 59)] and unable to pay their doctor bills

Meanwhile, Parisian hospitals overflowed, and "tent hospitals" were set up in people's yards and gardens (Figure 2.3). Half the inhabitants of Berlin were said to be infected.[4] It was everywhere. Yet, no one knew what caused it.

As bad as the Russian flu was, it was only moderate in severity com-pared to other influenza pandemics. Case fatality rates ranged from 0.1% to 0.28%, 10-fold lower than that of the deadly "Spanish" influ-enza pandemic of 1918. Its communicability was also moderate. The R0 (pronounced "R naught"; i.e., the median basic reproduction number of an infection) was estimated to be 2.1, meaning that, in a popula-tion of nonimmune people, each influenza case would subsequently infect 2.1 other individuals.[5] That number is comparable to the esti-mates in other flu pandemics, but considerably lower than for measles or chickenpox, the most contagious of human infections, with R0 of about 15 and 10, respectively.

Still, the Russian flu spread like rolling thunder, aided by crowding in the cities and by an increasingly interconnected world. Europe had more miles of railroads than it has today, and a trip across the Atlantic by ship averaged fewer than 6 days.[5] Further, by then, journalism was well established, and news of influenza and its impact on society cir-culated through the telegraph wires as fast as the illness itself. As with every epidemic, paralyzing fear of the infection traveled hand in hand with the disease itself. What was causing this terrible scourge?

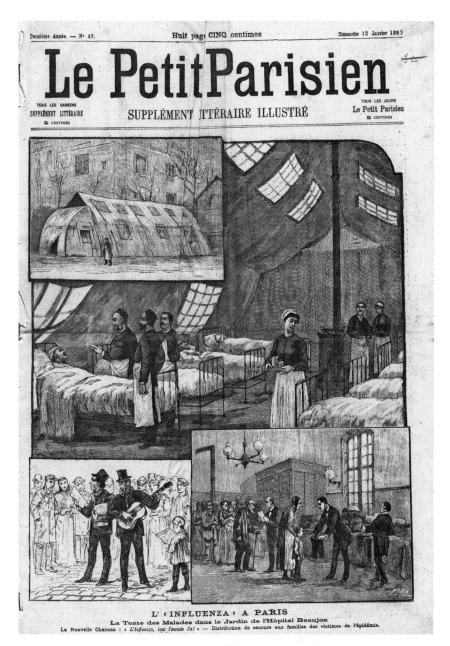

FIGURE 2.3 Magazine from 1890 depicting images of the Russian flu.

From US National Library of Medicine. The 1889 Russian Flu in the News. 2014, August 13. https://circulatingnow.nlm.nih.gov/2014/08/13/the-1889-russian-flu-in-the-news/

Even before the Common Era, scholars suspected the existence of tiny, invisible life forms and contemplated their roles in illness. In his treatise on agriculture, the Roman polymath Marcus Terentius Varro (116 BC to 27 BC) wrote the following advice regarding where to build a farmhouse:

> If you are forced to build on the bank of a river, be careful not to let the steading face the river, as it will be extremely cold in winter, and unwholesome in summer. Precautions must also be taken in the neighbourhood of swamps, both for the reasons given, and because there are bred certain minute creatures which cannot be seen by the eyes, which float in the air and enter the body through the mouth and nose and there cause serious diseases.[6](p. 209)

Recognition that microscopic organisms, rather than weather patterns or bad spirits or sinful acts, may cause disease subsequently led to the concept of disease transmission and contagion. In 1546 Girolamo Fracastoro, an Italian physician and poet, wrote of three types of contagion in his books *De Contagione et Contagiosis Morbis et eorum Curatione* [On Contagion, Contagious Diseases, and Their Cure].[7] The first was direct contagion, of which syphilis, known to be associated with sexual activity, was an example. Fracastoro detailed this in his poem "Syphilis sive Morbus Gallicus" [Syphilis or the French Disease]. Interestingly, that infection went by a number of names, including "the Polish sickness" by the Russians, "the German sickness" by the Poles, "the Neapolitan sickness" by the French, and "the Spanish sickness" by the Flemish, Dutch, Portuguese, and North Africans.[8] Fracastoro's second type of contagion was indirect through fomites, and he stated that wood or clothing (i.e., fomites) could transfer "seedlets of contagion" and thus spread infections. His third type was contagion at a distance, characterized by the spread of tuberculosis and smallpox, which seemed to fly through the air.

Many theories about the origin of influenza had been proposed through the centuries, and, during the Russian pandemic, as in earlier outbreaks, it was a hotly debated topic. By 1891, Dr. Henry Franklin Parsons concluded that "overcrowding and impure air" were powerful forces in propelling the epidemic and "poverty must have in many cases conduced to a fatal issue ... seeing that it often involves not only inferior conditions of lodgment, but also want of appropriate food, of sufficient warmth and clothing, and of ability to take the needed rest."[2(p. 107)]

Other scientists thought influenza came from Russian mud and most likely was due to a microbe called a strepso-bacillus (sic), while public health officials in England attributed it to a miasma, that is, a poisonous vapor arising from rotting matter. Parsons himself referred to the etiologic agent as a "poison."[2]

Establishing the cause of an infection can be tricky business. In 1832, 60 years before the Russian influenza pandemic, Charles Caldwell described the four elements of disease causation as (1) the remote, (2) the predisposing, (3) the occasional or exciting, and (4) the proximate, which succeeded one another, in that order, leading to illness. Caldwell gave an elusive example:

> The remote cause of bilious fever is malaria. That produces by its action on the system, a predisposition to the disease [bilious fever], which constitutes the predisposing cause. The exciting cause, acting on the body thus predisposed, produces the proximate cause, which, in the estimation of many, is the complaint itself.[9(p. 181)]

Caldwell further stated that

> measures for the prevention of disease are founded on a knowledge of its remote, predisposing, and exciting causes. Means of cure are instituted on an acquaintance with its proximate cause, a knowledge of which is attained, in part, from symptoms, but more certainly by post mortem inspection.[9(p. 182)]

This philosophy, complicated as it was, introduced to scientists and physicians a new way to think about the pathogenic mechanisms and etiologic factors that relate to disease.

As later explained by Dr. Richard Shope in reference to influenza,

> The remote cause was thought to be "some viscious [sic] quality of the air" and bore a relationship to the seasons and meteorological

conditions. The predisposing cause was defined as "that which renders the body liable or capable of being affected by disease when the exciting cause is applied." The exciting cause was considered to be "that external circumstance which kindles the fever, to wit, the morbid miasma, or contagion." The proximate cause, in reality probably an effect, was the inflammatory reaction in the respiratory tract responsible for the signs and symptoms of illness exhibited by the sick individual.[10(p. 417)]

These concepts fairly accurately describe the epidemiologic principles of an outbreak and the immune protection against infection. What was missing, though, in Caldwell's scheme of disease was knowledge of the actual microbial agent that caused the infection.

During the decade before the Russian flu appeared, important advances had occurred in the study of microbes, the tiny living organisms that could only be seen with a microscope. It was the so-called Golden Age of Bacteriology, and the most far-reaching advance was the growing acceptance of the germ theory of disease.[11] The bacteria that caused a number of infections, such as diphtheria, cholera, tuberculosis, anthrax, gonorrhea, typhoid fever, tetanus, and erysipelas (a skin infection), had been identified; methods for growing bacteria in the laboratory had been devised; and microscopes with high enough resolution to give fairly clear images of the bacteria had been developed. The microbes came in many shapes and sizes, some round, some long and thin, some twisty, some forked, all interesting (Figure 2.4). Maybe one of them caused influenza.

While people all over the world languished with the Russian flu, Dr. Richard Friedrich Johannes Pfeiffer, a curious physician in Berlin, peered into his microscope. He was gazing at a sputum specimen coughed up by a patient with Russian influenza. In the absence of influenza epidemics during the previous 40 years, very few patients had been available to study its etiology. Now that the disease was rampant, Pfeiffer seized the opportunity to learn what was causing such a widespread menace. Bacteria, those tiny creatures too little to see but too big to ignore, seemed a logical explanation.

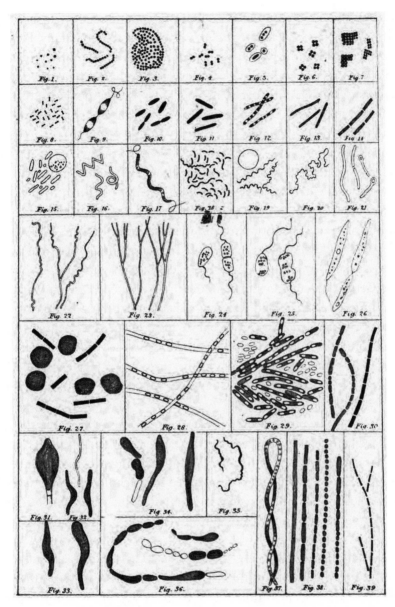

FIGURE 2.4 Drawings by Dr. Edgar Crookshank of the bacteria, "schizo-mycetes," and "fission-fungi." Pfeiffer's influenza bacillus was described after publication of this figure.

From Crookshank EM. *Manual of Bacteriology*. London: Lewis; 1889: Frontispiece.

Richard Pfeiffer, the son of Natalie Jüttner and Otto Pfeiffer, an educated but poor German clergyman, was born in 1858 in Zduny, Prussia (now Poland) and grew up in nearby Schweidnitz (now Swidnica, Poland). Limited family finances prevented Richard from attending a university, but he was an excellent student and won a spot at the Kaiser-Wilhelm Akademie, the prestigious Army medical school in Berlin. On graduation, he was assigned to a military station in Wiesbaden. A large typhoid fever outbreak swept through western Germany during his service there, and while trying to quell the infections, Pfeiffer became intrigued with microbes. He worked with a senior physician, A. Pfeiffer (no relation), and learned key bacteriology laboratory skills, such as how to accurately count bacteria in water samples.[12]

By 1887, Pfeiffer had been promoted to captain in the German army medical corps and was deployed to a backwater post in Lorraine during the German occupation that followed the Franco-Prussian War. He had little to do there and was very unhappy. It didn't take long, however, for his commanders to recognize his promise as a scientist. After only 2 months in dreadful Lorraine, he was assigned to assist the noted bacteriologist Dr. Robert Koch at the Institute of Hygiene at Berlin University (Figure 2.5). Pfeiffer certainly would have appreciated such a spectacular opportunity.

Koch, who would go on to receive the Nobel Prize in Physiology or Medicine, had high regard for the eager and gifted Pfeiffer. Under Koch's tutelage, and that of the other outstanding bacteriologists who had flocked to Berlin, Pfeiffer mastered the techniques of the day in microbiology, including using photomicroscopy, dissecting infected guinea pigs and pigeons, and culturing (i.e., propagating) bacteria on agar-containing dishes.

In 1891, four years after Pfeiffer joined Koch's laboratory, Koch named Pfeiffer director of the scientific section of the new Institut für Infektionskrankheiten [Institute of Infectious Diseases]. Since the Russian influenza pandemic was still raging through Europe, Pfeiffer, now able to work on his own research projects, set about to identify its cause.[12]

Pfeiffer's search for bacteria in the sputa from patients with influenza was based on the following observations: (1) Influenza occurred in pandemics; (2) influenza was contagious; and (3) influenza seemed to

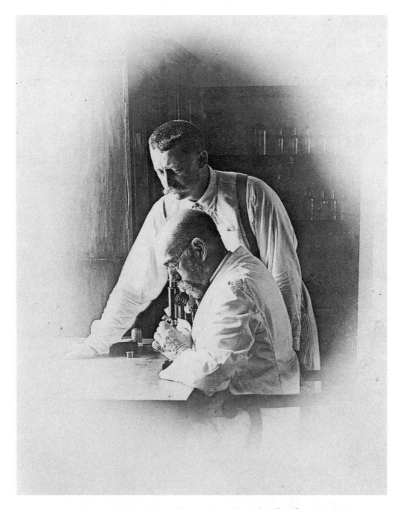

FIGURE 2.5 Robert Koch (seated) and Richard Pfeiffer working in a laboratory while investigating the plague in Bombay.
Courtesy of the Wellcome Trust Medical Library. Photograph attributed to Captain C. Moss, 1897.

spread via diseased secretions from patients.[13] Thus, he directed his attention to the respiratory secretions of influenza patients. He chose to study patients who produced large amounts of "well-compacted expectorations" and described the respiratory secretions in great and, to some readers, disgusting detail. They were yellowish-green, copious, viscous, and sticky. The patients coughed them up in "thick, coin-like clots."[13]

Through the lens of his microscope, Pfeiffer saw structures that looked like large quantities of bacilli (i.e., rod-shaped bacteria) nestled in the mucus (Figure 2.6). The bacilli were tiny, about the same thickness as mouse septicemia bacilli, which caused infections in mice, but only half their length. Sometimes three or four bacilli stuck together and formed a chain. Further, many were inside "pus cells."[13–15]

Pfeiffer had never seen bacteria that looked like these but he recognized them as possibly important. Thus, to better understand their pathogenic potential, he injected them into a variety of animals to see if they caused disease. Nothing happened to the guinea pigs, pigeons, rats, or mice he injected. Rabbits and monkeys, however, gave him "positive results"—whatever that meant; presumably the animals became ill. Because these microbes had come from patients with influenza, Pfeiffer—with less-than-complete scientific proof—took the bold step of announcing in a lecture in January 1892 to the Association of Physicians at the Charité hospital in Berlin that his newly described bacteria, the ones he called influenza bacilli, were the cause of influenza.[14]

Because he thought he had discovered the cause of influenza, Pfeiffer needed to better understand the influenza bacilli. His first challenge was

(a)   (b)

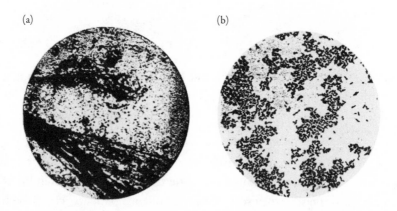

FIGURE 2.6 What Pfeiffer saw in the microscope. a, Sputum from a patient with severe pneumonia. b, Influenza bacilli in pure culture.

Adapted from Pfeiffer R. Die Aetiologie der Influenza [The Aetiology of Influenza]. *Zeitschrift für Hygiene und Infektionskrankheiten.* 1893;13:357–385.

to propagate the bacteria obtained from patient specimens. Without the ability to grow the microbes in his laboratory, he would be unable to study them extensively. Before the 1890s, gelatin had been used to thicken the laboratory fluids on which bacteria were cultured, but its lack of stability over wide temperatures caused great consternation among researchers. Bacteria that dipped and bobbed in soupy media were hard to tame.

About the time Pfeiffer was working with his newfound bacteria, Walther Hesse, one of Koch's assistants, spotted a row of his wife's freshly prepared jelly jars in their kitchen. He asked how the jellies remained firm during the heat of the summer. She explained a trick her mother had learned from an Indonesian neighbor in New York: the use of Japanese seaweed, called agar-agar, as a thickener.[16,17] Koch and his colleagues adopted its use but mentioned the technique for the first time, in passing, in his landmark paper describing the bacterial etiology of tuberculosis:

> The tubercle bacilli can also be found on other nutrient substrates when the latter have similar properties as solidified blood serum. For example, they grow on an agar-agar, prepared like permanently heat-hardy jellies, with an addition of meat and peptones. But they form, on this growth media, only small, irregularly shaped mounds, never as characteristic vegetations as in the blood-serum.[18(p. 225)] (Google translation)

Using the newly described solid medium with 1.5% sugar in agar, Pfeiffer was able to propagate his influenza bacteria in his laboratory, but he couldn't sustain their growth beyond one generation. His inability to keep them reproducing over many generations severely limited his potential to study them. Dr. Shibasaburo Kitasato, a widely recognized physician and scientist from Japan, was a visitor in Koch's laboratory at the time and couldn't understand why Pfeiffer's influenza bacilli hadn't been identified earlier, considering the hundreds of thousands people afflicted with influenza. Further, when hearing of Pfeiffer's difficulty growing the influenza bacilli, Kitasato thought the problem was that other, more rapidly growing, bacteria in the respiratory specimens outgrew the influenza bacilli.

Kitasato devised a method, similar to the one Koch used to study *Mycobacterium tuberculosis*, to cultivate Pfeiffer's bacteria on artificial media. Using glycerin agar, he let them grow for 10 generations, noting that, when grown on the agar, the little mounds of bacteria (i.e., the bacterial "colonies") looked like miniscule water droplets and were so tiny they were visible only with a magnifying glass. Kitasato agreed the organisms resembled no other bacteria previously grown from human infections.[19]

Pfeiffer struggled mightily to make his influenza bacilli survive beyond one generation on the agar dishes. He planted them on standard and glycerin agar and on gelatin, either at room temperature or in a warm incubator. He tried growing them in animal and human serum, bouillon, and milk, but nothing worked. Finally, he gave up trying to understand why Kitasato's method worked but his didn't, saying, "Maybe later investigators will be luckier."[13]

Ultimately, while trying to analyze why he had so much trouble growing the bacteria after the first generation, Pfeiffer surmised that because they grew well in patients' sputa, maybe the complex proteins, including blood, in respiratory secretions provided the necessary nutrients for growth. He then hypothesized that his bacteria might grow for several generations when cultured in blood. When he dropped human blood onto the agar plates, his bacteria, indeed, grew very well.[15] In fact, he was able to serially culture bacteria from a single specimen, over and over on blood-containing agar, for 8 months. Pfeiffer's breakthrough in growing the influenza bacilli in blood-containing artificial media not only permitted his research to move forward but also demonstrated to scientists who studied microbes the novel notion that specific bacteria require specific nutrients.

Pfeiffer had difficulty seeing his tiny new bacteria, even with the assistance of a microscope, especially when they were in small numbers. They looked a lot like the mucus and cellular debris in the sputum samples. In order to study them further, he needed to find a way to better visualize the influenza bacilli under the microscope.

Five years earlier, Hans Christian Gram, a Danish physician rather than a bacteriologist, had revolutionized the ability to visualize "schizomycetes," his word for bacteria. As the story goes, which may or may not be true, Gram was working in the morgue of the city hospital of Berlin, examining lung specimens from a patient who had died of pneumonia, when he inadvertently spilled iodine on methyl violet–stained lung specimens. He then tried to clean it up with alcohol. When he examined the specimens under the microscope, the bacteria in the lungs, which before the cleanup job had appeared purple, were now uncolored. Thus, he discovered that alcohol could wash away the purple stain from some bacteria that caused pneumonia, thereby distinguishing them from other bacteria that remained purple.[20]

Gram was a very modest man. In describing his staining method, he stated, "I am well aware that [my results] are brief and with many gaps. It is to be hoped that this method will also be useful in the hands of other workers."[21(p. 217)] His published paper was accompanied by a note from the editor of the journal, stating, "I would like to testify that I have found the Gram method to be one of the best and for many cases the best method which I have ever used for staining Schizomycetes."[21(p. 217)]

The editor was farsighted, as Gram's staining method remains a major initial step in identifying bacteria from clinical specimens. Knowing the Gram reaction and the microscopic morphology of yet-to-be-identified bacteria isolated from an ill patient gives a physician an important clue to the possible cause of the patient's illness. The physician can then prescribe initial, also called "empiric," antibiotic therapy that is likely to succeed in treating the infection based on whether the bacteria appear as rods (long and narrow) or cocci (round balls, like berries) and on their Gram reaction.

Pfeiffer attempted to stain his new bacilli using Gram's original method, which utilized crystal violet to tint the bacteria purple followed by alcohol treatment to decolorize them.[15] Unfortunately, the bacilli failed to stain purple, meaning Pfeiffer continued to have difficulty readily seeing them in sputum specimens. Much later, using the more contemporary Gram stain technique that added counterstaining with safranin, those bacilli, now called *Haemophilus influenzae*, would appear as delicate, blush-pink rods, sometimes in pairs, sometimes as singletons; sometimes they were very short and almost round, other times long and occasionally stringy. They are called pleomorphic, reflecting the many physical forms they may take.

Pfeiffer showed that his influenzal bacteria required oxygen to grow and did not grow at temperatures below 26°C or above 42°C. If kept under moist conditions on agar, the life span of the bacteria was 14 days. When he described the microscopic findings of the lungs of patients who died of influenza pneumonia, Pfeiffer noted the character of the pus as "reminiscent of [the discharge from] urethral and conjunctival gonorrhea," meaning that it was thick, gooey, and greenish-yellow. He elaborated on his earlier observation that blood facilitated the growth of influenza bacilli and demonstrated that, compared to blood from rabbits, guinea pigs, humans, or fish, the "growth was particularly lush" with pigeon blood.[13]

He wondered whether the influenza bacilli spread directly from person to person or by a "miasmatic path," such as through air, soil, or water. He demonstrated experimentally that his bacilli were extremely sensitive to drying and didn't survive in pure water. Based on these observations, he unequivocally stated, "With every sneeze, every cough these patients propel countless infectious germs into the environment from where they get, by breaths, into the respiratory organs of healthy individuals and infect them."[13]

When he finished his studies, Pfeiffer was more convinced than ever that he had discovered the etiology of influenza and titled the published scientific manuscript that described this more complete work *Die Aetiologie der Influenza* [The Etiology of Influenza]. In light of the photomicrographs Pfeiffer included in his paper and the state of the field of bacteriology at that time, he understandably thought the bacteria he saw in the sputa of influenza patients *must* be the cause of influenza.

Pfeiffer's proclamation that influenza bacilli were the cause of influenza was heralded as the most important scientific advance of the epidemic.[22] Most physicians embraced his proclamation. But, was it correct?

In an attempt to systematize causation of infectious diseases, Pfeiffer's mentor, Robert Koch, developed criteria to establish the etiologic relationship between bacteria and wound infections. Later, he applied these principles to anthrax, cholera and tuberculosis.[23] These criteria, known as "Koch's postulates," established in 1878, fourteen years before Pfeiffer's proclamation that influenzal bacilli caused influenza, stated

1. Infected tissue must show the presence of a particular microorganism not found in healthy subjects;
2. The microorganism must be isolated and grown in a pure culture;
3. When injected into a healthy animal, the microorganism must cause the disease associated with it; and
4. The "second-generation" microorganism should then be isolated and shown to be identical with the microorganism found in the first postulate.[24,25]

These postulates, which have been updated to incorporate modern scientific methods and concepts, remain the essential framework for establishing the bacterial etiology of infectious diseases.[26] They define causation as demonstrating

1. The bacteria under study are present in all diseased subjects and absent in healthy persons.
2. The bacteria can be cultured in the laboratory with no other bacteria present in the specimen.
3. The bacteria cause disease in animals that is similar to the disease in humans.
4. Bacteria isolated from infected animals are identical to those isolated from the human specimen as detailed in Postulate 1.

When the postulates are met, scientists are willing to accept that a bacterium isolated from an infected patient truly represents the cause of the infection.

Did Pfeiffer's bacilli meet Koch's postulates? In his papers, Pfeiffer clearly documented, in photomicrographs, that his bacilli obtained from the respiratory tracts of patients with influenza grow in pure culture in the laboratory (meaning no other bacteria grew from the specimen), thus meeting Koch's second postulate. When Pfeiffer injected rabbits with his bacilli, they did not develop the symptoms of classic human influenza, but, rather, developed high fever, as did many patients with influenza.[13] Thus, a case could be made that these results at least partially fulfilled Koch's third postulate. The purulent material from the experimental rabbits' bronchi contained bacteria in pure culture very similar to Pfeiffer's bacilli isolated from patients with influenza, thus meeting Koch's fourth postulate.

Koch's first postulate—infected tissue must show the presence of a particular microorganism not found in healthy subjects—was the hardest to prove. Pfeiffer didn't clearly document the inclusion of sputa from healthy people in his studies. Microbiologists in that era had not yet recognized that bacteria living normally on the mucosal surfaces, such as the airways, of healthy people can be both human pathogens (those that cause disease, such as pneumonia, in the lung) and commensals (those that live in human throats without causing disease). This circumstance, known as colonization, threw an interfering flying object into Koch's postulates when trying to apply them to Pfeiffer's bacillus as the cause of influenza.

Although in his postulates Koch alluded to the use of experimental controls, they were not common in scientific experimentation at that time. Dr. John Snow, famously credited with identifying water as the source of the cholera epidemic in London in 1855, observed that the number of cases decreased significantly after he removed the handle from the Broad Street pump, but he didn't investigate the number of healthy people without cholera who received water from that pump, nor the number of cholera patients who never used that pump. That controlled experiment was done by a local London minister in the same year.[27] Valid controls were not routinely included in published studies until the 1920s,[28] and case-control studies did not become standard experimental practice until after the 1950s, when they were successfully incorporated into studies linking cigarette smoking with cancer.[29]

In spite of general enthusiasm for Pfeiffer's proclamation that influenza bacilli caused influenza, his proclamation raised nagging doubts among some bacteriologists.[30,31] For starters, Dr. David Davis pointedly noted that Pfeiffer's original paper was "singularly free from statistical detail. He does not state how many cases he examined nor the percentages of positive and negative results by cultural methods. He uses general expressions such as 'the bacilli were always found in sputum, etc.'"[32]

In the decade after Pfeiffer first declared that his bacilli caused influenza, a number of other scientists also isolated his bacteria from patients with influenza, seemingly confirming Pfeiffer's proclamation.[33] When Davis inoculated his own nose and tonsils with a large dose of the bacteria (early bacteriologists often used themselves to study human infections), he developed mild fever, cough, and a sore throat with thick mucus on his pharyngeal wall from which large numbers of Pfeiffer's bacilli were cultured. To his surprise, cultures from his throat remained positive for those bacilli for a month.[34]

Other studies, however, contradicted Pfeiffer's proclamation. In one, his bacilli were isolated from 92% of patients with whooping cough but from only 18% of patients with influenza. Further, the bacilli were also isolated from the throats of a few patients with chickenpox, measles, pertussis, and tuberculosis and, importantly, from children with meningitis.[35] These observations suggested that Pfeiffer's bacilli were "saprophytes," harmless colonizers present in the respiratory tracts of healthy people, with the possible potential of somehow changing into a pathogen that causes influenza.[36]

Pfeiffer, convinced his influenza bacilli caused the respiratory disease influenza, focused his studies exclusively on infection in the lungs. Other investigators found that, in addition to being isolated from sputum samples of patients thought to have influenza, influenza bacilli could also be isolated from the cerebrospinal fluid that bathed their brains.[37-40] Thus, such patients were thought to have meningitis as a component of their influenza infection, and the meningeal infection was thought to be caused by whatever had caused the influenza. The question remained: What caused influenza?

For three decades, Pfeiffer's bacillus was accepted as the cause of influenza because no other credible cause had been found.[41-43] It remained the best, albeit disputed, explanation until the Spanish influenza pandemic of 1918–1919, which provided thousands of cases for careful bacterial analysis. In most of those studies, Pfeiffer's bacilli were isolated from some, but certainly not all, influenza patients and were isolated from patients with other infectious diseases, thus violating Koch's first postulate of causation.[44]

The variability in finding influenza bacilli in influenza patients was, probably accurately, attributed in part to variations in laboratory techniques, for these bacteria were, and still are, notorious for their "fastidious" nature, meaning they are persnickety in the laboratory and refuse to grow on ordinary agar under ordinary culture conditions. Pfeiffer had shown that nutrients mattered, that the growth media had to include blood for his bacteria to grow, but not all blood was equal. Sheep's blood, commonly used in making routine blood agar, contains an enzyme that interferes with growth of the influenza bacillus, whereas rabbit and horse blood actively, and human blood only moderately, supported growth.[45]

While Pfeiffer himself referred to his bacteria as influenza bacilli, other early investigators called them *Bacillus influenzae* in keeping with the scientific taxonomy convention for naming biologic creatures.[35,37] They have a first name and a last name, always written in italics.[46] The first is the genus (group) name, and the second (more specific) is the species name, for example, *Homo sapiens, Homo neanderthalensis,* and *Homo erectus,* which denote modern man, early man, and even earlier hominids, respectively[47]; and *H. influenzae* and *Haemophilus parasuis,* which denote a pathogen of humans and pigs, respectively. The genus and species names of bacteria may reflect the names of scientists, such as *Salmonella typhi* in honor of Dr. Daniel Salmon; the place of discovery, such as *Providencia stuartii* for Providence, Rhode Island; the disease associated with the bacteria, such as *Vibrio cholera*; or a particular characteristic of the bacteria, such as *Streptococcus viridans* for the green halo around the colonies grown on blood agar (enzymes from the streptococci diffuse into the agar and partially degrade the hemoglobin in the surrounding red blood cells into methemoglobin, which metabolizes to green pigments).[48] Thus, *Bacillus influenzae* (abbreviated *B. influenzae*) was named for the shape of the bacteria (bacillus or rod) and for the disease it was thought to cause (influenza).

Scientists strive for order; thus, living things are organized into the major domains of life: Bacteria, Eukarya, and Archaea. This hierarchical scheme, based on the organization of their genetic material, then further clusters alike creatures together in order to distinguish them from unalike creatures, similar to the scheme originally described by Ernst Haeckel in which bacteria fell into the Protista kingdom (the other two were Plantae and Animalae) (Figure 2.7).[49] In today's taxonomy, bacteria are grouped into stratified clusters,

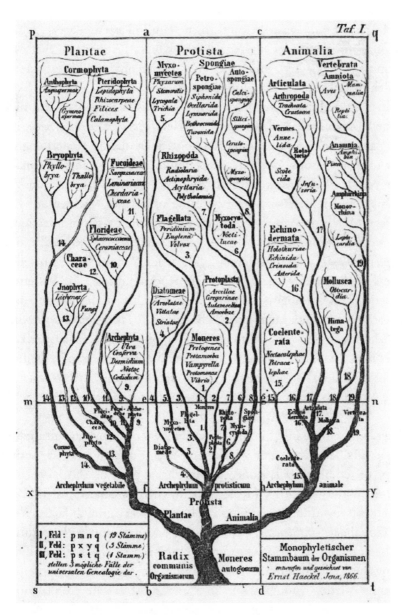

FIGURE 2.7 Haeckel's tree of life. Bacteria would fall into the Protista column.

From Haeckel E. *Generelle Morphologie der Organismen* (Vol. 2). Berlin: Reimer; 1866:465.

such that *H. influenzae* belongs to the family Pasteurellaceae, which belongs to the order Pasteurellales, which belongs to the class Gammaproteobacter, which belongs to the phylum Protobacteria, which belongs to the kingdom Bacteria.

In 1897, Lehmann and Newmann, the first scientists to chronicle bacterial taxonomy, called Pfeiffer's bacteria *Bacterium influenzae*, but the name *Bacillus influenzae* seemed to stick among the bacteriologists. For unclear reasons, in their compendium Lehmann and Newmann grouped *B. influenzae* with both *Mycobacterium leprae* (the cause of leprosy) and *Bacterium pestis* (the cause of plague),[50] which are very different kinds of bacteria that cause very different types of infections.

Bacillus influenzae had other names, including *Pyobacillus* and *Diplobacillus*,[51] as well as hemophilic bacillus[35] and Pfeiffer's bacillus, terms used by many scientists in their reports. In 1917, the Society of American Bacteriologists' committee on the characterization and classification of bacterial types officially named it *Hemophilus influenzae*, based on its need for blood to grow.[51] The genus name *Hemophilus* derives from the Greek *haima* = "blood" and *philos* = "lover."[52] Pfeiffer's bacillus, indeed, loved blood. More recently, the British spelling *Haemophilus* is used by most scientists for the species designation.[53(p. xv)]

After he discovered that influenza bacilli grew better when cultured on blood, Pfeiffer investigated which components of blood, namely serum alone or red blood cells alone, facilitated that growth. The answer was the red corpuscles. After further experiments, he determined that the hemoglobin within the red blood cells was the key growth factor.[13]

Why did *H. influenzae*, but not other bacteria, require the addition of hemoglobin to the agar to grow? The answer was iron. All living things need iron to survive. But free iron is very toxic to cells, so rather than percolating through tissues in its raw, noxious state, iron is bound to proteins (e.g., iron-containing heme, which combines with the globin protein to form hemoglobin), thus allowing the iron to circulate and nourish the body's cells and yet insulate them from the metal's toxicity. Hence, iron in the form of heme is available to human cells for their metabolic needs without damaging human tissues.

Bacteria also require iron for their metabolic processes, and most manufacture their own protective protein, heme, from complex molecular building blocks. This process requires a number of enzymes. *Haemophilus influenzae* is unique among bacteria in that it lacks six of the seven enzymes needed to make heme. As a workaround, *H. influenzae* steals the penultimate building block protoporphyrin IX from the body of the person in which the bacteria live and then uses the bacteria's lone heme enzyme, ferrochetolase, to act on the stolen protoporphyrin IX to complete the process of manufacturing heme.[54] The glycine agar that Pfeiffer used to grow the influenza bacillus, the same agar he and Koch used to grow other bacteria they studied, didn't have protoporphyrin IX in it, so the *B. influenzae* couldn't make its own heme and thus wouldn't grow. Only when he added blood, and with it the iron-containing heme in the red cells' hemoglobin, did his bacteria thrive.

Subsequently, *B. influenzae* was defined by its need for two specific nutrients, called "vitamins," to grow.[55] One was hemoglobin, as Pfeiffer had found, which was ultimately called X factor.[56] The other was present in yeast and in plant material and was called V factor. Later, V factor was identified as coenzyme nicotinamide adenine dinucleotide (NAD),[57] which is necessary for survival of all living cells as it is required for a number of biochemical processes.

The same year that Pfeiffer first identified *B. influenzae* (1892), a botanist in Russia showed that mosaic disease of tobacco could be spread from plant to plant by a transmissible agent capable of passing through filters that trapped bacteria.[58] With that discovery, entirely new life forms, eventually known as viruses, were shown to be agents of illness, and the field of virology was born. Subsequently, many scientists began using filters to study the nature of infections that didn't appear to be caused by bacteria. During the Spanish flu pandemic of 1918, filtered sputum from an influenza patient was injected into two healthy people, and the subjects developed symptoms of influenza.[59] In addition, a scientist sprayed his and his technician's throats with filtered throat washings from several influenza patients, and they both developed mild influenza symptoms, suggesting a filterable agent, rather than *B. influenzae*, caused influenza.[60]

The word *virus* comes from the Latin *virus*, meaning slimy liquid or poison, and originally referred to snake venom.[1] From the early

1700s to the early 1920s, it meant a morbid principle or poisonous substance produced in the body. In the 1800s, it began to connote an infectious, usually submicroscopic, principle of disease that could be inoculated into another person to cause that disease. By 1929, a virus was considered to be a filterable disease-causing agent, meaning that it was not trapped by the filters used by bacteriologists at that time. Ultimately, based on accumulated knowledge, it has come to mean a DNA- (or RNA-) containing infectious agent that multiplies only within the cells of living hosts. Most recently, the meaning of virus includes a malicious software program that infects computer systems.

Not everyone, however, believed the results suggesting influenza was caused by a filterable agent because (1) small numbers of experiments were performed; (2) quarantine procedures were not in place to ensure the subjects didn't get influenza from their friends, relatives, or neighbors; and (3) the incubation period between instillation of the filtrate and appearance of symptoms was variable.[61] Further, other investigators who inoculated volunteers with filtered sputa obtained different results.[44,62] A major step forward in identifying the true cause of influenza came in 1920 when rabbits, infected by Peter Olitsky and Fredrick Gates with filtered sputa from influenza patients, developed an illness similar to the infection caused by inoculation with unfiltered sputa, thus strongly suggesting that bacteria, which would be trapped in the filters, were *not* the cause of influenza.[63]

For the next decade, scientists demanded definite proof that a filterable agent caused influenza, but the experimental results did not always support such a hypothesis. Meanwhile, viruses became well recognized as causing human disease, and laboratory techniques were developed to study them. At the same time that the 1918 Spanish influenza pandemic appeared in humans, a new illness resembling human influenza was recognized among hogs in several midwestern states.[62] Veterinarians called it swine flu. In 1931, the virologist Richard Shope published a series of papers documenting the cause of swine influenza as the influenza virus in combination with *Hemophilus influenzae suis* (now called *H. parasuis*), a pathogen of young pigs that is very similar to *H. influenzae*.[10] Studies that followed in humans and ferrets (the best animal model for influenza) successfully fulfilled Koch's postulates[64,65] and established without a doubt that influenza virus was the true cause of influenza.

For decades, scientists puzzled over which influenza virus was actually responsible for the Russian pandemic. Finally, in 2014, phylogenetic techniques (examining evolutionary patterns of the virus genes) and seroarcheologic techniques (measuring antibodies likely present in people at various points in time) were applied to the question of which virus caused the Russian flu of 1889–1892. The results showed that it was likely caused by influenza type A virus, whose hemagglutinin (one of the proteins on the surface of the virus) was of the H3 type and whose neuraminidase (an enzyme of the surface of the virus) was of the N8 type.[66]

Thus, Pfeiffer's proclamation that his bacillus caused influenza was finally proven wrong. His identification of *B. influenzae* in the respiratory tract, however, was a major contribution to the scientific understanding of bacterial infections and moved the field of bacteriology forward in allowing other investigators to unearth its full potential as an important human pathogen. Further, in the course of his studies of *B. influenzae*, Pfeiffer pioneered the field of nutritional requirements of bacteria. Finally, Pfeiffer's identification of *H. influenzae* launched subsequent studies of the causes of bacterial meningitis and initiated in-depth explorations of bacterial meningitis-causing pathogens that ground our concepts of pathogenesis, and guide our management, of the infection.

After his identification of *B. influenzae*, Pfeiffer went on to make additional important scientific discoveries. He accompanied his former mentor Robert Koch to India to investigate an outbreak of plague and to Italy, where he studied malaria. He contributed to the identification of the respiratory pathogen *Mikrococcus catarrhalis* (now called *Moraxella catarrhalis*). He recognized that bacteria, when exposed to serum, broke apart and died, thus establishing the role of serum in mediating immunity against many bacteria, such as those that cause cholera, pneumonia, and meningitis.[12] And, he introduced the concept of "endotoxin" to describe the toxic component of *V. cholera*.

Endotoxins are complex molecules of sugars (polysaccharides) and fats (lipids) present in the membranes surrounding many gram-negative bacteria. Or as Pfeiffer described it, endotoxin is "the bacterial body sub-stance" responsible for the symptoms of septic shock during an infec-tion. When Pfeiffer infected guinea pigs with cholera bacteria, he found that the toxic effects of the bacteria, as mediated by the "bacterial body substance" did not depend on living bacteria.[67] This was a revolutionary concept at the time, and, as subsequent research confirmed Pfeiffer's re-sults, this observation won him accolades as the "father of endotoxin."[68]

During his studies of malarial parasites, Pfeiffer became frustrated with the images produced by standard microscopes. They were inverted, so everything appeared upside down compared to the true image. Building on his skills in photomicrography, he modified the micro-scope built by Ernst Leitz so it provided an erect image (Figure 2.8).[69] This improvement allowed scientists to see the correct orientation of

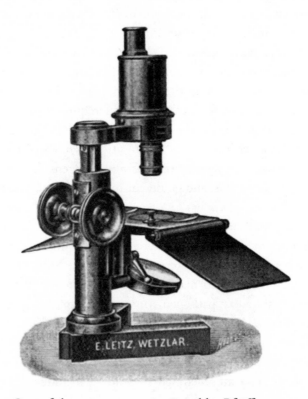

FIGURE 2.8 One of the microscopes invented by Pfeiffer.

From Bennett AW, ed. Pfeiffer's New Preparation Microscope. *Journal of the Royal Microscopical Society.* 1900, p. 509.

the object they were viewing, rather than resorting to mentally turning an upside-down image to right side up or, worse yet, turning the microscope front to back in order to view the image. For his excellence as an investigator, Pfeiffer was elected a Foreign Member of the British Royal Society in 1928.

In writing Pfeiffer's memoir, the bacteriologist Paul Fildes, Pfeiffer's friend and admirer, described him as having "uttered hard words about scientific opponents and, indeed, his writings show that he would not stand any nonsense. But, he was always polite." Further, "he must have been a man of authority, but he certainly did not use this gift to further any ambitions outside his scientific work. He is said to have been indifferent to honours." This altruism likely contributed to his calming influence on his temperamental mentor, Robert Koch.[12] Pfeiffer was recognized by his peers as a meticulous researcher—supported by the experimental detail in his publications—who was forceful and persistent in defending his scientific work. In papers published in 1922 and 1925, well after most scientists accepted a virus as the cause of influenza, he expressed skepticism of the value of "the refined methods of modern microbiology" (meaning the new world of viruses) and continued to support his notion that *B. influenzae* caused influenza.[70,71] The proud man just wouldn't give it up.

Pfeiffer's most meaningful scientific discoveries were made while he worked with Koch; he published 34 papers between 1892 and 1896. After he left Berlin, first to become chairman of hygiene in Königsberg (now Kaliningrad, Russia) and a decade later chairman of hygiene in Breslau (now Wrocław, Poland), he focused his academic efforts on teaching until he retired in 1926 at age 68 (Figure 2.9). By then the world was changing around him. World War I had taken a terrible toll on his country and National Socialism was rising in Germany. Pfeiffer had been educated by the German army and, as a young man, served as a military officer. Yet, he found the growing Nazism distasteful. In 1933, his former student and valued colleague Carl Prausnitz was arrested, likely because his father was half-Jewish. In 1939, at age 81, Pfeiffer moved to the bucolic little resort town of Bad Landeck (now Lądek Zdrój) in Poland, on the present-day border with Czechoslovakia, where he had often gone on vacation.[12]

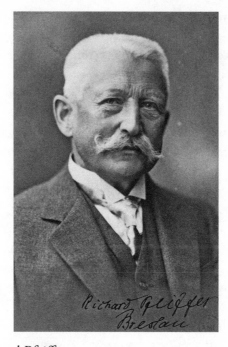

FIGURE 2.9 Richard Pfeiffer.
From https://commons.wikimedia.org/wiki/File:Richard_Pfeiffer.jpg (US public domain image).

The historical record is, for the most part, silent on Pfeiffer's personal life, other than information from his longtime, loyal maid, Frau Hedwig (Hedel) Köhler, from Bad Landeck.[12,72] Pfeiffer's wife, Elizabeth Teubner, whom he married in 1891,[73] died in 1934. In 1939, he married his wife's niece, with whom he shared a love of music; she was an opera singer and he an amateur composer and accomplished pianist with a passion for Beethoven and Chopin.[72] His second wife died of gastric cancer a year after their marriage. For the rest of his life, despite suffering from gout and senile atherosclerosis, he enjoyed working in his garden, reading, editing a German microbiology journal, and taking daily walks with Frau Köhler to the Forest Cemetery.

Although Pfeiffer escaped much of the turmoil of World War II, the liberating Russians arrived in Bad Landeck in May 1945, and most German residents fled to the west. Pfeiffer reportedly refused to leave.

After the Russian soldiers decamped, his quiet little house was subsequently conscripted to billet Polish soldiers, described as "satellite Poles" as they remained loyal to the Soviet regime, and Pfeiffer was confined to one room on the second floor, one story above both his beloved piano and his bed. On September 15, 1945, at age 87, a broken and lonely man, he died and, and according to Frau Köhler as reported by Fildes, was buried in the churchyard of the Bad Landeck parish church.[12]

References

1. Simpson J, Weiner E. *Oxford English Dictionary*. Oxford, England: Oxford University Press; 1996.
2. Parsons HF. *Report on the Influenza Epidemic of 1889–90*. London: HM Stationery Office; 1891.
3. Smith FB. The Russian Influenza in the United Kingdom, 1889–1894. *Social History of Medicine*. 1995;8(1):55–73.
4. Kempińska-Mirosławska B, Woÿniak-Kosek A. The Influenza Epidemic of 1889–90 in Selected European Cities—A Picture Based on the Reports of Two Poznań Daily Newspapers from the Second Half of the Nineteenth Century. *Medical Science Monitor*. 2013;19(Dec 10):1131–1141.
5. Valleron A-J, Cori A, Valtat S, Meurisse S, Carrat F, Boelle P-Y. Transmissibility and Geographic Spread of the 1889 Influenza Pandemic. *Proceedings of the National Academy of Sciences of the United States of America*. 2010;107(19):8778–8781.
6. Cato MP, Varro MT. *Marcus Porcius Cato, On Agriculture; Marcus Terentius Varro, On Agriculture*. Cambridge, MA: Harvard University Press; 1934.
7. Nutton V. The Reception of Fracastoro's Theory of Contagion: The Seed That Fell Among Thorns? *Osiris*. 1990;6:196–234.
8. Rothschild BM. History of Syphilis. *Clinical Infectious Diseases*. 2005;40(10):1454–1463.
9. Caldwell C. Thoughts on the Causes of Disease, More Especially the Predisposing Cause, with Practical Remarks. *Transylvania Journal of Medicine and the Associate Sciences*. 1944;23:415–455.
10. Shope RE. Old, Intermediate, and Contemporary Contributions to Our Knowledge of Pandemic Influenza. *Medicine*. 1944;23(4):415–455.
11. Blevins SM, Bronze MS. Robert Koch and the Golden Age of Bacteriology. *International Journal of Infectious Diseases*. 2010;14(9):e744–e751.
12. Fildes P. Richard Friedrich Johannes Pfeiffer. 1858–1945. *Biographical Memoirs of Fellows of the Royal Society*. 1956;2(Nov 1):237–247.
13. Pfeiffer R. Die Aetiologie der Influenza. *Zeitschrift für Hygiene und Infektionskrankheiten*. 1893;13:357–385.

14. Pfeiffer R. Vorläufige Mittheilungen über die Erregerder Influenza. *Deutche Medizinische Wochenschrift.* 1892;18(2):28.

15. Pfeiffer R, Beck M. Weitere Mittheilungen uber den Erreger der Influenza. *Deutche Medizinische Wochenschrift.* 1892;18(21):465.

16. Hesse W. Walther and Angelina Hesse—Early Contributors to Bacteriology. *ASM News.* 1992;58(8):425–428.

17. Hitchens AP, Leikind MC. The Introduction of Agar-Agar into Bacteriology. *Journal of Bacteriology.* 1939;37(5):485–493.

18. Koch R. Die Aetiologie der Tuberkulose. *Berliner klinische Wochenschrift.* 1892;19(15):221–230.

19. Kitasato S. Aus dem Institut für Infektionskrankheiten III. Ueber den Influenzabacillus und sein Culturverfahren. *Deutsche Medizinische Wochenschrift.* 1892;18(2):28.

20. Casanova JM. Bacteria and Their Dyes: Hans Christian Joachim Gram. *Immunologia.* 1992;11(4):140–150.

21. Brock TD. *Milestones in Microbiology 1546 to 1940.* Washington, DC: ASM Press; 1999.

22. Leichtenstern OML. *History, Epidemiology, and Etiology of Influenza.* Philadelphia: Saunders; 1905.

23. Centers for Disease Control. Historical Perspectives Centennial: Koch's Discovery of the Tubercle Bacillus. *MMWR Morbidity and Mortality Weekly Report.* 1982;31:121–123.

24. Koch R. *Untersuchungen über die Aetiologie der Wundinfectionskrankheiten.* Leipzig: Vogel; 1878.

25. Special Article on Immunity II. *Journal of the American Medical Association.* 1905;44(5):389–391.

26. Fredericks DN, Relman DA. Sequence-Based Identification of Microbial Pathogens: A Reconsideration of Koch's Postulates. *Clinical Microbiology Reviews.* 1996;9(1):18–33.

27. Cholera Inquiring Committee. *Report of the Cholera Outbreak in the Parish of St. James, Westminster, During the Autumn of 1854.* London: Churchill; 1855.

28. Morabia A. Snippets from the Past: Is Flint, Michigan, the Birthplace of the Case-Control Study? *American Journal of Epidemiology.* 2013;178(12):1687–1690.

29. Paneth N, Susser E, Susser M. Origins and Early Development of the Case-Control Study: Part 1, Early Evolution. *Sozial-und Praventivmedizin.* 2002;47(5):282–288.

30. Fildes P, McIntosh J. The Aetiology of Influenza. *British Journal of Experimental Pathology.* 1920;1(2):119–126.

31. Mathers G. The Bacteriology of Acute Epidemic Respiratory Infections Commonly Called Influenza. *Journal of Infectious Diseases.* 1917;21(1):1–8.

32. Davis DJ. The Bacteriology of Influenza. *Proceedings of the Institute of Medicine of Chicago.* 1919;2:142–150.

33. Eyler JM. The State of Science, Microbiology, and Vaccines Circa 1918. *Public Health Reports.* 2010;125(Suppl 3):27–36.

34. Davis DJ. The Bacteriology of Whooping Cough. *Journal of Infectious Diseases.* 1906;3(1):1–37.

35. Davis DJ. Influenzal Meningitis. *Archives of Internal Medicine.* 1909;4(4):323–329.

36. Emery Wd'E. The Micro-organisms of Influenza. *Practitioner.* 1907;78(1):109–117.

37. Holt LE. Observations on Three Hundred Cases of Acute Meningitis in Infants and Young Children. *American Journal of Diseases of Children.* 1911;1(1):26–36.

38. Wollstein M. Influenzal Meningitis and Its Experimental Production. *American Journal of Diseases of Children.* 1911;1(1):42–58.

39. Dunn CH. Cerebrospinal Meningitis, Its Etiology, Diagnosis, Prognosis and Treatment. *American Journal of Diseases of Children.* 1911;1(2):95–112.

40. Davis DJ. Influenzal Meningitis, with Especial Reference to Its Pathology and Bacteriology. *American Journal of Diseases of Children.* 1911;1(4): 249–265.

41. Jordan EO, Falk IS. *The Newer Knowledge of Bacteriology and Immunology.* Chicago: University of Chicago Press; 1927.

42. Cecil RL, Blake FG. Studies on Experimental Pneumonia X. Pathology of Experimental Influenza and of *Bacillus influenzae* in Monkeys. *The Journal of Experimental Medicine.* 1920;32(6):719–752.

43. Blake FG, Cecil RL. Studies on Experimental Pneumonia IX. Production in Monkeys of an Acute Respiratory Disease Resembling Influenza by Inoculation with *Bacillus influenzae*. *The Journal of Experimental Medicine.* 1920;32(6):691–718.

44. Taubenberger JK, Hultin JV, Morens DM. Discovery and Characterization of the 1918 Pandemic Influenza Virus in Historical Context. *Antiviral Therapy.* 2007;12(4 Pt b):581–591.

45. Krumwiede E, Kuttner AG. A Growth Inhibitory Substance for the Influenza Group of Organisms in the Blood of Various Animal Species. *The Journal of Experimental Medicine.* 1938;67(3):429.

46. Hardy J. *Naming Conventions: Nomenclature of Microorganisms.* 2011. http:// hardydiagnostics.com/wp-content/uploads/2016/05/nomenclature-of-microorganisms.pdf. Accessed July 28, 2017.

47. Smithsonian National Museum of Natural History. *What Does It Mean to be Human?* 2018. http://humanorigins.si.edu/evidence/human-fossils/species. Accessed December 18, 2018.

48. Gooch JW. Alpha (α) Hemolysis. In: Gooch JW, ed. *Encyclopedic Dictionary of Polymers.* New York: Springer; 2011:873.

49. Haeckel E. *Generelle Morphologie der Organismen.* Berlin: Reimer; 1860.

50. Lehmann KB, Neumann RO. *Atlas and Essentials of Bacteriology.* New York: Wood; 1897.

51. Winslow C-EA, Broadhurst J, Buchanan RE, Krumwiede C, Rogers LA, Smith GH. The Families and Genera of the Bacteria: Preliminary Report of the Committee of the Society of American Bacteriologists on Characterization and Classification of Bacterial Types. *Journal of Bacteriology.* 1917;2(5):505–566.

52. Kilian M. Genus III. Haemophilus In: Brenner DJ, Krieg NR, Staley JT, eds. *Bergey's Manual of Systemic Bacteriology* (Vol. 2). New York: Springer; 2005:883.

53. Sell, SH, Wright, PF. Haemophilus influenzae: *Epidemiology, immunology, and prevention of disease.* New York: Elsevier; 1982.

54. White DC, Granick S. Hemin Biosynthesis in *Haemophilus. Journal of Bacteriology.* 1963;85(4):842–850.

55. Davis DJ. Food Accessory Factors (Vitamins) in Bacterial Culture with Especial Reference to Hemophilic Bacilli I. *The Journal of Infectious Diseases.* 1917;21(4):392–703.

56. Thjotta T, Avery OT. Growth Accessory Substances in the Nutrition of Bacteria. *Experimental Biology and Medicine.* 1921;18(6):197–199.

57. Lwoff A, Lwoff M. Studies on Codehydrogenases, I. Nature of Growth Factor "V." *Proceedings of the Royal Society of London Series B.* 1937;122(5):352–359.

58. Ivanowski D. Concerning the Mosaic Disease of the Tobacco Plant. In: *Phytopathological Classics* (Vol. 7). St. Paul, MN: American Phytopathological Society; 1968:27–30.

59. Nicolle C, Charles L. Quelques Notions Expérimentales sur le Virus de la Grippe. *Comptes Rendus de l'Académie des Sciences.* 1918;167(Oct 14):607–610.

60. Selter H. Zur Aetiologie der Influenza. *Deutsche medizinische Wochenschrift.* 1918;44(2):932–933.

61. Dochez AR, Mills KC, Kneeland Y. Studies on the Virus of Influenza. *The Journal of Experimental Medicine.* 1936;63(4):581–598.

62. Shope RE. Recent Knowledge Concerning Influenza. *Annals of Internal Medicine.* 1937;11(1):1–12.

63. Olitsky PK, Gates FL. Experimental Study of the Nasopharyngeal Secretions from Influenza Patients: Preliminary Report. *Journal of the American Medical Association.* 1920;74(22):1497–1499.

64. Smith W, Andrewes CH, Laidlaw PP. A Virus Obtained from Influenza Patients. *The Lancet.* 1933;222(5732):66–68.

65. Francis T. Transmission of Influenza by a Filterable Virus. *Science.* 1934;80(2081):457–459.

66. Worobey M, Han G-Z, Rambaut A. Genesis and Pathogenesis of the 1918 Pandemic H1N1 Influenza A Virus. *Proceedings of the National Academy of Sciences of the United States of America.* 2014;111(22):8107–8112.

67. Pfeiffer R. Untersuchungen über das Choleragift. *Zeitschrift für Hygiene.* 1891;11:393–411.

68. Rietschel ET, Cavaillon JM. Richard Pfeiffer and Alexandre
    Besredka: Creators of the Concept of Endotoxin and Anti-endotoxin.
    Microbes and Infection. 2003;5(15):1407–1414.

69. Summary of Current Researches Relating to Zoology and
    Botany: Microscopy. *Journal of the Royal Microscopical Society.*
    1890;10(4):501–541.

70. Pfeiffer R. Das Influenzaproblem. *Ergebnisse der Hygiene, Bakteriologie,
    Immunitätsforschung und experimentellen Therapie.* 1922;5(1):1–18.

71. Pfeiffer R. Neuere Forschungen zur Klärung der Influenzaätiologie. *Deutsche
    medizinische Wochenschrift.* 1925;51(1):10–13.

72. Kathe J. In Memoriam: Richard Pfeiffer. *Zentralblatt für Bakteriologie,
    Parasitenkunde, Infektionskrankheiten und Hygiene 1 Abt, Originale.*
    1958;171(4–5):217–223.

73. Gerabek WE. Pfeiffer, Richard Friedrich Johannes. *New German Biography.*
    2001. https://www.deutsche-biographie.de/pnd116163895.html#ndbcontent_
    werke. Accessed February 3, 2016.

3

On Immunity

EVEN DURING ANCIENT TIMES, certain societies understood protective immunity, the ability of the body to resist microbial infection. They recognized that some illnesses attacked a person once and then never again. They also knew how to shield themselves from the evils of several diseases by exposing themselves to weakened substances related to the disease. Pliny the Elder claimed that the snake-charming Psylli people of North Africa didn't succumb to snakebites because they drank water from wells inhabited by snakes. Further, the Nobel Prize–winning physiologist Emil von Behring described a tribe in Mozambique whose members protected themselves from fatal snakebites by rubbing a paste containing snake venom into small skin incisions.[1] In addition, "inoculation of the smallpox virus"—virus here means a generic infectious agent, as true viruses hadn't been discovered yet—by mixing it with milk and injecting it under the skin of the arm had been "practiced by the Burmese from time immemorial" to prevent smallpox.[2,3(p. 48)]

One of the first well-documented reports that employed the concept of immunity emerged from the plague of Athens during the Peloponnesian War, which pitted the Spartans against the Athenians. Between 430 and 426 BCE, an illness characterized by the sudden onset of severe headache followed by fiery red eyes, throat, and tongue stormed through the Athenians. Cough followed, then abdominal pain and bilious vomiting. The patients felt feverish, and their skin was "reddish, livid, marked all over with little pustules and sores" (or a rash of

Continual Raving: A History of Meningitis and the People Who Conquered It. Janet R Gilsdorf, Oxford University Press (2020). © Oxford University Press.
DOI: 10.1093/oso/9780190677312.001.0001

some kind). Many died, and some who lived lost their eyes, their extremities (presumably from gangrene), or "all memory."[4(p. 229)]

The nature of the plague of Athens has been debated through the ages; smallpox, typhoid fever, Ebola, measles, and typhus have all been implicated on the basis of the clinical signs and the epidemiology of known infectious diseases.[5–8] The suggestion of typhoid fever as the cause, based recently on *Salmonella typhi*–like DNA found in the teeth pulp from a mass gravesite at the ancient Kerameikos cemetery of Athens, has been disputed because the investigators didn't include dirt from the gravesite as a control.[9] Irrespective of the actual cause, the Athenian general and historian Thucydides, who himself had the disease, commanded survivors to care for their sick friends and family members, as he recognized that, even with intense exposure, those who survived the highly contagious plague of Athens did not experience a second episode.[10]

In the tenth century, the Chinese protected their children from smallpox by drying the gooey scab from a smallpox sore, covering it with cotton, and shoving it into the nostrils of those who had not yet been infected; they called the process "sowing the Small Pox."[11(p. 15)] Subsequently, the smallpox inoculation procedure spread to India and Africa. In Constantinople in the early eighteenth century, inoculation was performed by scratching the material from a smallpox sore into the skin of children. On learning of this practice, Lady Mary Wortley Montagu, the wife of the British ambassador to Turkey, became a strong advocate of the procedure (Figure 3.1).

A witty and elegant socialite, Lady Montagu, herself, had contracted smallpox at age 26, three years after her marriage to Sir Wortley Montagu, and suffered facial scarring as a result. In one of her poems, "Smallpox,"[12] she described a previously beautiful woman as she looked into her mirror after recovering from the disease:[13]

> How am I chang'd ! alas ! how am I grown
> A frightful spectre, to myself unknown !
> Where's my Complexion? where the radiant Bloom,
> That promis'd happiness for Years to come?[12]

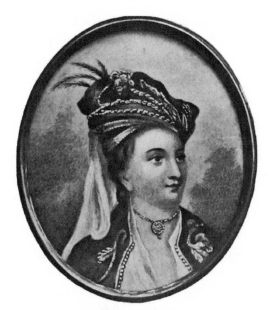

LADY MARY WORTLEY MONTAGU
FROM A MINIATURE

FIGURE 3.1 Lady Mary Wortley Montagu.
From Paston G. *Lady Mary Wortley Montagu and Her Times*. London: Putnam's; 1907:242ff.

When she returned to England in 1721, Lady Montagu introduced variolation, or inoculation, against smallpox—the disease was also called variola—to western Europe. As she wrote in one of her letters, she hoped her friend Mrs. S. C. would admire her heroism as she proceeded to push her discovery—inoculation to prevent smallpox—on British doctors.[14] She adamantly insisted that Dr. Charles Maitland inoculate her own daughter, aged 2 years old, against the disease.[15]

Variolation came to America through African slaves; the Puritan minister Cotton Mather in Massachusetts learned of the practice from his slave, Onesimus, who had been vaccinated as a child in his homeland, likely what is now Ghana.[16,17] Mather then read details of the inoculation procedure in the *Philosophical Transactions of the Royal Society* and persuaded Dr. Zebdiel Boylston to perform the procedure on the people of Boston.[11,18,19] Although the European royalty had eagerly embraced variolation,[20] the technique didn't immediately catch on in the

United States because the protection it provided was variable, and the procedure sometimes resulted in severe smallpox infection with occasional death.[21] Immunity to smallpox, and the freedom from infection it afforded, came with a cost.

The word *immunity* rose from the Latin *immunis*, which means to be free, exempt from public service, or exempt from a tribute.[22] An early use of the term as a medical word by David Craigie referred to protection against yellow fever: "Previous to the year 1793, a degree of immunity [against yellow fever] ... had been enjoyed by most of the West India colonies and the towns of the United States for a space of at least ten years."[23(p. 229)] The author, as well as other physicians, attributed yellow fever immunity to the "electrical" characteristics of the atmosphere, citing as evidence that the islands of the West Indies exhibiting "fresh winds, gales, hurricanes, and tornadoes" were less affected by the disease than the other islands. This, of course, was wrong. Immunity has nothing to do with the weather.

By 30 years later, the understanding of the nature of immunity hadn't progressed much. Dr. William Ogle inferred possible mechanisms of diphtheria immunity from his observations of the hygiene in the homes of his diphtheria patients who resided in rural English villages where that disease was relatively rare. He suggested that to protect children against the disease, the following hazards, which he had seen only in the households of the infected, should be avoided: (1) highly offensive, untrapped grates leading to the main sewer; (2) overflowing, filthy privies; (3) open cesspools and pig sties; and (4) accumulation of fecal matter behind wainscots.[24] The world hadn't yet learned that the spread of diphtheria is not related to fecal contamination, but rather is spread from person to person by respiratory droplets, with no animal or environmental intermediary.[25]

In addition, Ogle, who was the medical officer of health for a rural district of England, had witnessed second episodes of the disease in several of his patients and noted "that no perfect immunity can thus be acquired is certain." Yet, he also stated that he had little doubt "that some degree of protection is conferred by an attack against future ones."[24(p. 714)] By this he implied the diphtheria infection bestowed partial, or imperfect, immunity against subsequent diphtheria infections.

By 1903, awareness of the mechanisms of immunity remained limited. Dr. William Ainley-Walker recognized that some members of any animal species, including humans, were more susceptible to certain infections than others were or, as he said, were "more predisposed."[10(p. 169)] He then explained predisposition as the converse of immunity and considered immunity to be relative rather than absolute as it could be diminished by "anemia, deprivation of water, dyscrasias [disorders] of the blood, fatigue, nerve-poisons [whatever they were], extirpation of organs, general diseases [such as diabetes], bad food, and many other causes."[10(p. 170)] Thus, immunity didn't always offer complete protection and, indeed, could be modified, or compromised, by a variety of interfering medical, or other, conditions.

In setting the stage for his treatise on immunity, Ainley-Walker alluded to Charles Darwin's theory of evolution in that animals predisposed to infection, either through heredity or by acquired means, may become infected with bacteria and then succumb to the resultant disease.[10] Thus, the more highly susceptible animals would die and fail to propagate, while the less susceptible (i.e., immune) would escape the infection. To him, the natural action of infections was to improve the "physical standard" of the species by "the survival of the fittest," meaning that immunity to infection led to well-being in both individual animals and the population at large. In a little dig at his own profession, Ainley-Walker stated that in humans, this process is "continually thwarted by the efforts of the physician, whose duty is to preserve the unfit for as long as possible."[10(p. 169)]

As a British country doctor, Edward Jenner traveled from farm to farm caring for his patients and observed that horses were subject to a disease the farriers called "the Grease." This illness was characterized by "inflammation and swelling of the heel, from which issues matter possessing properties of a very peculiar kind which seems capable of generating a disease in the Human Body, which bears [a] strong a resemblance to the Small Pox." He also observed a servant, "not paying due attention to cleanliness," move from applying dressings over the diseased heels of the horses to milking the cows, with "some particles of the infectious matter adhering to his fingers." Jenner deduced, then, that thus the "disease is communicated to the Cows, and from the Cows to the Dairymaids."[26(p. 3)]

Further, when he tried to inoculate dairy folk with smallpox, often they failed to develop the characteristic sore with surrounding redness that indicated the inoculation had been successful. Therefore, grease in the horses → cowpox in the cattle → cowpox in the milkmaids → protection of the milkmaids from smallpox inoculation. Jenner found it remarkable that, "in the present age of scientific investigation ... a disease of so peculiar a nature as the Cow Pox ... should so long have escaped particular attention."[26(p, iii)]

While cowpox sores on people looked like smallpox sores, they were considerably fewer in number, generally appeared only on an infected person's hands and wrists, and didn't lead to scarring, to severe disease, or to death as smallpox often did. Rather, infection with cowpox resulted in fever and headache for several days, and then the sores slowly healed. Jenner further stated, "What renders the Cow-pox [*sic*] virus [virus here is generic for an infectious agent] so extremely singular is that the person who has been thus affected is forever-after secure from the infection of the Small Pox."[26(p. 6)] Thus, cowpox conferred immunity to smallpox on the dairy workers.

One of Jenner's patients, the milkmaid Sarah Nelms, developed cowpox on her hand at the site of a previous scratch from a thorn (Figure 3.2). On May 14, 1796, seeking "the more accurately to observe the progress of the infection," Jenner scraped debris from the sores on Sarah Nelms's hands and inoculated it into the arm of 8-year-old James

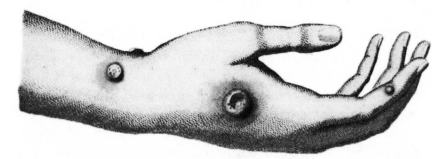

FIGURE 3.2 Cowpox lesions on Sarah Nelms's hand.

From Jenner E. *An Inquiry into the Causes and Effects of the Variolae Vaccinae, a Disease Discovered in Some of the Western Counties of England, Particularly Gloucestershire and Known by the Name of Cow Pox.* London: Sampson Low; 1798:32ff.

Phelps through two incisions, each ½-inch long and barely penetrating the skin. A week later, James had discomfort in his armpit, and 2 days after that, felt chilly, lost his appetite, and had a slight headache. After a restless night, he felt fine the next day. Jenner reported that the healing of James's cowpox variolation sore progressed to a scab (dried blood) and then to an eschar (a scab with dead tissue in it) in a similar fashion as that of a sore from inoculation with smallpox matter.[26]

To prove the efficacy of his cowpox variolation procedure to protect against smallpox, 2 months later, on July 1, 1796, Jenner inoculated James Phelps again, but this time he used material from a fresh smallpox sore. James did not become ill. Several months after that, Jenner repeated the smallpox injection and, again, James remained well.

In his scientific report, which was self-published as a monograph, Jenner described 23 "cases" of cowpox or inoculation of cowpox matter from person to person (Figure 3.3) and concluded, "I shall myself continue to prosecute this inquiry, encouraged by the hope of its becoming

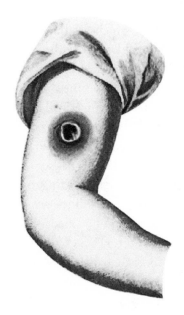

FIGURE 3.3 Cowpox variolation scab on Jenner's patient 18.

From Jenner E. *An Inquiry into the Causes and Effects of the Variolae Vaccinae, a Disease Discovered in Some of the Western Counties of England, Particularly Gloucestershire and Known by the Name of Cow Pox.* London: Sampson Low; 1798:32ff.

essentially beneficial to mankind."[26(p. 75)] The cowpox variolation method had worked to protect vaccinees against smallpox and was much safer than smallpox variolation. What wasn't known, though, was *how* it worked. That knowledge would come much later.

The word *smallpox* emerged in the seventeenth century to distinguish the disease from syphilis, which was called pockes or pockys or pox.[27] Thus, syphilis, first widely recognized by the generalized, pustular lesions characteristic of secondary syphilis, was called the great pox, and the disease caused by what we now know as variola virus was called the lesser, or small, pox. Cowpox referred to similar sores on the udders of cows. Chickenpox was named for the resemblance of its lesions to chickpeas[28] and is caused by a virus unrelated to cowpox or smallpox.

The virus that has most recently been used in smallpox vaccines is neither cowpox nor variola (smallpox) virus, but, rather, is a different, but related, orthopox virus called vaccinia. The genetic relationships between these three viruses are complicated and not completely understood. Phylogenetic studies that analyze the relatedness of their genes suggested that cowpox virus, which has the widest host range (rodents, cats, cattle, humans[29]) is the oldest of the three.[30] Between the time that Jenner injected James Phelps with the cowpox virus from Sarah Nelms's hand and the time that smallpox vaccines became regulated, a number of cowpox viruses from different sources had been passed repeatedly between humans, from which standardized strains began to be used for vaccination. As the viruses were thus passed from person to person, population bottlenecks occurred such that subsequent surviving viruses displayed more limited gene diversity, leading to the theory that vaccinia and variola evolved from cowpox, with the accompanying loss of genes through reductive evolution. Another theory suggests vaccinia is actually a derivative of horsepox virus, which is the largest of the orthopox viruses.[31] This theory is consistent with the association between the disease grease in horses and cowpox in cattle.[32] Thus, the true genetic ancestry of the vaccinia virus is complex and hidden in the veil of time.[33]

Immunity against smallpox through vaccination has been the most successful of any immunization strategy to date, as smallpox has been eradicated from Earth because of widespread immunization. This feat of immense magnitude was accomplished by unprecedented global public health efforts. The last wild-type case of smallpox occurred in 1977 in a Somali man named Ali Maalin.[5] Today, the only known remaining smallpox viruses reside in secure public health facilities at the State Research Centre of Virology and Biotechnology (VECTOR) in Koltsova near Novosibirsk (in Siberia), Russia, and at the Centers for Disease Control and Prevention in Atlanta, Georgia, in the United States.[34] Other samples may unknowingly exist, however; in 2014 a cardboard box containing six vials of variola was found in a cold storage room owned by the Food and Drug Administration and located at the National Institutes of Health in Washington, D.C.[35]

During the late 1800s and early 1900s, a war of words raged among physicians and scientists regarding the nature of immunity: Some supported the so-called cellular theory and others the serum, or humoral, theory. Considerable laboratory research was mounted by scientists on each side to refute the findings of those on the other.[36] The cellular theory was championed by Élie Metchnikoff, a Russian zoologist at the Pasteur Institute in Paris, who first described the antibacterial action of neutrophils, the phagocytic white blood cells that ingest and digest bacteria.[37] The serum theory, fostered by the German scientists George Nuttall, W. von Grohmann, and Hans Buchner, focused on the ability of serum (the liquid remaining after blood has clotted) or plasma (the liquid component of blood after the cells have been removed by centrifugation), both lacking neutrophils, to kill a variety of bacteria.[38] The unknown factor in the serum responsible for the bacterial killing was originally called alexine.[39]

These two camps, the cell theory people and the serum (or humoral) theory people, passionately clung to their respective beliefs and sometimes lobbed disrespectful comments, or downright insults, very publicly at each other. Buchner, during a lecture in Munich, stated,[40] "The presence of [bacterial killing] action in body fluids reveals the overall detectable activity of phagocytes as less decisive," and, in response, Metchnikoff wrote, "the postulates of this [serum] theory are often not in accord with the real facts. ... Alexine is nothing but a leukocytic product."[37(p. 184)]

The German bacteriologist Carl Flügge (whom Metchnikoff snidely called "the learned Breslau hygienist") disliked Metchnikoff's notion of bacteria being eaten by human cells and wrote, "There is no . . . analogy between the ingestion of food and the struggle against infective micro-organisms, nor between nutritive substances and living micro-organisms."[37(p. 525)]

Metchnikoff devoted over 20 pages in his book to arguing his case, writing, "The attempts of the partisans of the [bacterial killing] theory of the body fluids have failed whenever it was necessary to give evidence of their action in the refractory animal."[37(p. 184)] It eventually devolved into a fight about French science versus German science.

A major blow to Metchnikoff's cell theory was research conducted by Dr. Richard Pfeiffer, the German physician who discovered *Bacillus influenzae*. Pfeiffer injected bacteria that cause cholera into the abdomens of guinea pigs immune to cholera and saw that the bacteria swelled, dissolved, and disappeared within 20 minutes, too soon for phagocytic cells to have wandered into the tissues.[41] During the course of these experiments, however, when Pfeiffer mixed the bacteria with heated immune serum in test tubes, they didn't swell and die as they had in infected guinea pigs. He predicted that anticholeral factors in the immune serum were somehow modified when they were inside the animals, and the modification, whatever it was, promoted the serum-mediated killing that he so beautifully demonstrated in the animals. The world took notice of Pfeiffer's results, and for several decades, scientists, who referred to it as "Pfeiffer's phenomenon," considered it interesting, probably important, but mysterious. Although he didn't completely understand the mechanisms inside the animals underlying the bacterial killing that hadn't been apparent in the test tube, Pfeiffer had unwittingly observed the action of the guinea pig's own serum protein, complement, which, in concert with the immune serum, promoted killing of the cholera bacteria in the animals.

Ultimately, both theories, the killing power of serum and the phagocytic activity of the leukocytes, were recognized to be operative in immunity because they work together, like the strings (phagocytic cells) and the horns (serum killing factors) that meld with the other instruments (various immune factors) in an orchestra (the body) to facilitate a rich, complete, albeit complex, immune response.[42] Indeed, the same year that Ainley-Walker published his review paper acknowledging the importance of both serum and cells, Wright and Douglas published a paper describing cell-serum interactions. In it, the authors described a process they called opsonization, stating,

> We have here conclusive proof that the blood fluids [serum] modify the bacteria in a manner which renders them a ready prey to the phagocytes. We may speak of this as an "opsonic" effect (opsono—I cater for, I prepare victuals for), and we may employ the term "opsonins" to designate the elements in the blood fluids which produce this effect.[43(p. 366)]

Little by little, the scientists began to recognize the components of serum that served as opsonins to facilitate the ability of phagocytes to ingest bacteria (Figure 3.4).

While other scientists heatedly argued the nature of immunity, Dr. Martha Wollstein, the pediatric pathologist in New York who had described the clinical features of *B. influenzae* meningitis, labored steadily in her laboratory and in the autopsy suite at Babies' Hospital. As children on the hospital's wards died of meningitis, she toiled to understand what made those infections so deadly. She was one of the

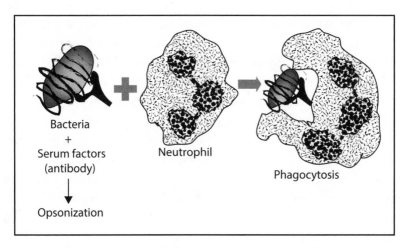

FIGURE 3.4 Opsonization and phagocytosis. Antibodies bind to bacteria, leading to opsonization, by which neutrophils ingest the antibody-bacterium complexes.

Drawing by the author.

few pathologists committed to understanding the illnesses of children and studied mumps, dysentery, and the pathological aspects of pneumonia, as well as the pathophysiology of pneumococcal infections. She is, however, best known for her studies of *B. influenzae*, which she lovingly described as "dew drop colonies" when grown on agar, and for their role in immunity and meningitis.[44]

Wollstein was a quiet woman. In her obituary in the *American Journal of Diseases of Children*, she was described as a person with "a modest, retiring disposition, [who] avoided public demonstrations and speechmaking as far as possible, but with those who sought her help as man to man [*sic*], she eagerly shared her wide store of knowledge with open generosity."[45(p. 1301)]

Born in November 1868 to Jewish immigrants from Germany, Wollstein and her five siblings (Edward, Adolph, Isaac, Rose and Helene) grew up in New York City, where their wealthy parents, Louis and Minna (Cohn) Wollstein, ran several businesses, including textile manufacturing,[46] cigar lighter manufacturing,[47] and gold refining.[48,49] She attended the Woman's Medical College of the New York Infirmary, established in 1868 to provide medical training to women who weren't allowed to attend established medical schools. In 1889, the year the Russian influenza pandemic began, Wollstein received her medical degree. She chose to forgo clinical practice and trained in infectious diseases research at the Rockefeller Institute and later continued her research studies as a pediatric pathologist at Babies' Hospital.[50]

In 1911, Wollstein wrote a paper describing eight cases of influenzal meningitis in children ages 5 months to 4 years. All of the cases were fatal. As a pathologist, she didn't provide clinical care for these patients, but focused her work on the blood and spinal fluid specimens that had been sent to her and on the *B. influenzae* that had caused the infections.[51] Motivated by the extremely high fatality rate of influenzal meningitis, she modeled her research on the work of her colleagues at the Rockefeller Institute, particularly that of Dr. Simon Flexner, who developed immune serum against epidemic meningitis (caused by what is now called *Neisseria meningitides* or meningococci).

Wollstein was eager to expand Flexner's findings to other bacteria that cause meningitis, particularly Pfeiffer's bacilli, so she initiated studies to follow the course of experimental influenzal meningitis in monkeys, which would serve as a proxy for studying the course of the infection in humans. She began by identifying the most virulent *B. influenzae* strains to use for her experiments and documented that those bacteria, indeed, caused meningitis in monkeys. Further, she established that the nonhuman primate disease was pathologically similar to the illness she had seen in humans. Then she injected a large number of live *B. influenzae* into the subdural spaces within the meninges of the monkeys' lumbar spines and set about studying immunity and its ability to prevent meningitis.[52]

Wollstein's work built on the understanding of immunity at that time. Four forms were recognized[10]:

1. Natural immunity, which originally was thought to be an inherited characteristic but we now know develops after a person is exposed to, and develops an immune response to, molecules commonly found in nature that are similar to those on microbes;
2. Passive immunity, which resulted from infusing serum that contained protective immune factors into a nonimmune animal or person;
3. Active immunity, which occurred after active infection or inoculation (e.g., smallpox variolation); and
4. Inherited immunity, a unique form of passive immunity in which immune protection is transferred from an immune mother, via her own serum antibodies that traverse the placenta, to her baby.[22]

At the time that Wollstein was conducting her research with *B. influenzae*, other scientists at the Rockefeller Institute were investigating the ability of passive immunity to treat meningitis caused by other bacteria. This treatment scheme was built on the profoundly important earlier studies of von Behring and Kitasato (the same Kitasato from Japan who had worked with Richard Pfeiffer on the discovery of *B. influenzae*) that revealed the mechanism of vaccine protection. Von Behring and Kitasato immunized rabbits with toxic proteins, or toxins, of the bacteria that cause tetanus and diphtheria, harvested the resulting immune sera from the animals, and injected it into mice. When the mice were challenged with tetanus- and diphtheria-causing bacteria, the mice were protected from infection and remained well.[53] Similarly,

Wollstein repeatedly immunized a goat with live *B. influenzae*, and the resultant goat immune serum, when injected into other animals, protected mice against *B. influenzae* blood infection[52] and protected monkeys against *B. influenzae* meningitis.[54] Something in the goat immune serum mediated the protection from infection.

The active immunity that Wollstein produced by immunizing the goat with *B. influenzae* was described by Louis Mitchell as occurring when

> the invaded organism [an infected animal or person] possesses the power of annulling or neutralizing the toxicity of bacterial poisons by virtue of the elaboration of antidotal substances through the agency of its living cells. These protective bodies appear in the animal juices, notably the blood-serum, and several of them are now known. ... Substances which appear during spontaneous or artificial infection or intoxication are known as antibodies and antitoxins.[55(p. 231)]

Among the first to use the term *antibodies* was Dr. Richard Pfeiffer when he wrote, in German, of *antikorpern*, which translates as "antibodies," to describe the factors in horse immune serum that protected against cholera in his experiments.[41]

While studying human immunity against bacteria, Richard Pfeiffer and his colleague Wilhelm Kolle immunized human volunteers with the bacteria that cause typhoid fever and cholera and demonstrated that the inoculations protected the recipients against each disease, respectively.[56,57] Further, when the immune serum was mixed with the bacteria in test tubes, the bacteria clumped together, and the degree of the clumping correlated with the ability of the immune serum to protect against disease. Much later, the mechanism of the clumping would be determined: Each antibody molecule in the serum attached to two bacteria, which resulted in a lattice of antibodies plus bacteria that was seen as clumps in the test tube. They looked like the gently falling flakes inside a snow globe. The clumping was termed *agglutination*, and the antibodies that resulted in clumping were called *agglutinins* (Figure 3.5).

When examining *B. influenzae* under the microscope, Wollstein noted the irregular morphology of the bacteria that had been cultured on

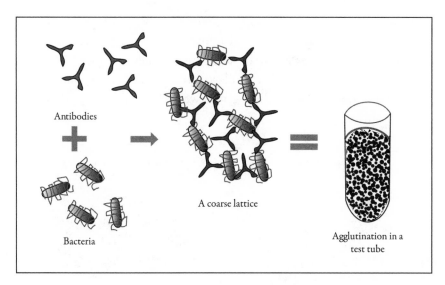

FIGURE 3.5 Agglutination reaction. Antibodies bind to bacteria, forming a lattice, which appears as clumping in the liquid environment of a test tube.

Drawing by the author.

agar—some were long, some short, and some thicker than others. The shapes of the bacteria correlated somewhat with their virulence in animals: Meningitis strains were longer and thicker and more virulent in rabbits than shorter, thinner respiratory strains. She was curious to know if these different morphoforms reflected different immunologic characteristics of the bacteria. She set out to answer that question by employing the serologic techniques available to her at the Rockefeller Institute: agglutination, complement fixation, opsonization, and immune protection against infection.[44]

To perform her studies, she produced immune sera by immunizing rabbits with *B. influenzae* isolated from either meningitis or respiratory specimens. When she mixed the rabbits' immune sera with *B. influenzae*, the bacteria clumped, evidence that the rabbit blood contained antibodies to that bacterial strain. The agglutination reactions, however, were weak and showed no strain specificity, that is, immune sera made from all the bacterial strains clumped all the bacteria to at least some degree. These results suggested all *B. influenzae* strains were immunologically alike. She examined the immune sera for complement fixation, which is the ability of the bacteria-antibody complexes to bind complement, the component of serum that, in the presence of antibodies, punches holes in the bacterial membranes and thus kills them (Figure 3.6).[58] These results, similar to the agglutination results, suggested no immunologic differences between the strains.

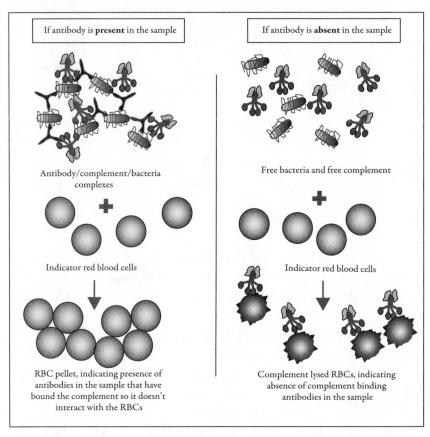

FIGURE 3.6 Complement fixation reaction. If complement is present in the reaction, antibody-bacteria complexes bind to the complement, and, when mixed with the red blood cells, the red cells clump and remain intact, indicating that the antibody-bacteria complexes have bound, or "fixed," complement. If complement is absent in the reaction, antibody-bacteria complexes that haven't bound to, or fixed, complement bind to red blood cells and lyse them. RBC, red blood cell.

Drawing by the author.

Wollstein's next experiments examined the rabbit immune sera for the presence of opsonins, those factors in blood that enhance the ability of neutrophils to engulf and digest bacteria as first described by Wright and Douglas.[43] When she mixed the immune sera with *B. influenzae* and then added neutrophils, she noted phagocytosis, but, again, the reaction showed no strain specificity: The immune sera prepared from all the *B. influenzae* strains opsonized all bacterial strains.

Finally, she performed the premier test of immunity—animal protection—to determine the ability of a previous infection to protect rabbits against repeat infection by a different bacterial strain. She infected rabbits with respiratory strains of *B. influenzae* and later challenged the rabbits with injections of meningitis strains and watched for illness in the animals. The results were inconsistent; sometimes the rabbits were protected from illness, sometimes not. Thus, Wollstein could not distinguish *B. influenzae* strains from each other immunologically and concluded they belonged to only one serologic class.

In 1919, the role of *B. influenzae* in the disease influenza was still a question among many scientists, so Wollstein performed additional serologic tests to try to sort it out. She obtained immune serum from patients who had recently had influenza and tested their sera for agglutination of *B. influenzae* (the results were poor) and for complement fixation (the results were irregular) and showed no difference between respiratory and meningitis *B. influenzae* strains. She introduced a new serologic test, the precipitation reaction, in which she broke apart the influenzal bacteria and mixed the bacterial fragments in a test tube with immune serum from patients. The antibodies in the serum, which were called "precipitins," attached to the little pieces of the bacteria, resulting in haziness that looked like morning mist in the test tube (Figure 3.7). Thus the serum from the patients contained precipitating antibodies, but, like the complement-fixing antibodies, there was no difference between reactions using respiratory or meningitis *B. influenzae* strains.[59]

In animal protection experiments, Wollstein observed that while her rabbit immune serum protected mice against *B. influenzae* infection, the sera from patients who had recently had influenza did not. Therefore, after using all the serologic tools available to her, the best Wollstein could say was the following:

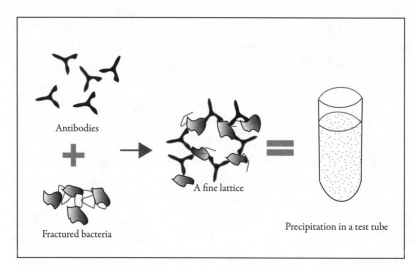

Antibodies

A fine lattice

Fractured bacteria

Precipitation in a test tube

FIGURE 3.7 A precipitation reaction. Antibodies bind to fractured bacteria, forming a fine lattice of antibody-bacteria complexes; the lattice appears as a fine mist in the liquid environment in a test tube.
Drawing by the author.

> The patients' serological reactions indicate the parasitic nature of the bacillus [*B. influenzae*], but are not sufficiently stable and clean-cut to signify that Pfeiffer's bacillus is the specific inciting agent of epidemic influenza. They do, however, indicate that the bacillus of Pfeiffer is at least a very common secondary invader in influenza, and that its presence influences the course of the pathological process.[59(p. 568)]

In reading her published reports, one can sense her extreme, albeit understated, frustration with the results of her immunology experiments, as they were confusing and impossible to interpret. It was a big disappointment for such a careful scientist. The tests she performed using immune sera developed from different strains of *B. influenzae* did not reveal immunologic differences among the strains. Meningitis strains generated stronger immune reactions and produced more intense disease in rabbits than respiratory strains, and yet, at that time, Pfeiffer's bacillus was still thought to cause influenza, a respiratory infection, and meningitis was thought to be a complication of influenza. Because Wollstein thought the respiratory strains and meningitis

B. influenzae strains were all related to the same disease process, she didn't understand why they should look different under the microscope, show different virulence characteristics when injected into rabbits, and yet appear to be immunologically similar in her experiments. She was definitely on the right track, but the key finding, to be discovered a bit later by Dr. Margaret Pittman, wasn't available to her yet.

Two years after her appointment as head of the pediatric section of the New York Academy of Sciences, Wollstein became the first woman admitted to the American Pediatric Society, the leading association of researchers in pediatrics.[50] During her career she authored over 80 scientific papers that focused on a variety of infectious diseases, including meningitis, diarrhea, malaria, tuberculosis, and typhoid fever.

In spite of her unassuming nature, Wollstein was a strong supporter of women in medicine and wrote often about Dr. Elizabeth Blackwell, the first woman to be granted a medical degree in America and founder of the Woman's Medical College of the New York Infirmary. In her comprehensive article, "The History of Women in Medicine," Wollstein emphasized the important role of women healers through the ages. She told of the curative incantations of the priestesses of ancient Greece and Egypt and of Isolda of Ireland, who sailed off to become the queen of Cornwall, bearing a chest of drugs ranging from love philters to death potions. She wrote of eleventh-century doctresses connected to the Salerno school of medicine and of Saint Hildegarde of Germany who authored two works of anatomy and physiology. In concluding, Wollstein paid homage to her own research interests, stating, proudly, "That women are particularly well adapted to laboratory work has always been admitted."[60] Dr. Simon Flexner, one of her mentors, may not have agreed with that sentiment, as he reportedly failed to give her the respect he gave to others, who were all men, in his research group,[61] and she failed to be elected to membership in the Rockefeller Institute.[62]

Wollstein was described as difficult to work with, had few known close friends, and "formed no close bonds with either sex."[62] Further, in the 1910 US census, when she was 41 years old, she is listed as living with her parents, a 15-year-old niece, and two servants. She retired in 1935 to Grand Rapids, Michigan, and maintained a home in Flushing,

New York, where she died in 1939 at the age of 70. She is buried in Beth El Cemetery in Queens, New York.[63]

Apparently family tensions plagued the Wollsteins. Her father's obituary notice in *The New York Times* stated that he left only a dollar each to his two oldest sons (Adolph and Edward) because their whereabouts were unknown. He didn't even know whether they were alive or dead.[64] Martha, though, must have been good to her parents, for in her father's will she received the family art, furniture, jewelry, and several life insurance benefits, as well as a third of the family home. Helene and Isaac received less.

Unfortunately, her important contributions to infectious diseases— her pioneering studies, albeit with confusing results, of immunity against *B. influenzae* and her early clinical descriptions of *B. influenzae* meningitis—were unknown among nonmedical folks and were quickly forgotten among her medical colleagues. Her very brief obituary in *The New York Times*, October 31, 1939, stated that, besides being a retired New York physician, she "was also known as a pathologist."[65]

References

1. Special Article on Immunity IV. *Journal of the American Medical Association.* 1905;44(6):475.
2. Gould GM. Medical Discoveries by the Non-Medical. *Journal of the American Medical Association.* 1903;40(22):1477–1487.
3. Macdonald KN. *The Practice of Medicine Among the Burmese:* Translated from original manuscripts, with an historical sketch of the progress of medicine from the earliest times. Edinburgh: MacLachlan and Stewart; 1879.
4. Thucydides. *History of the Peloponnesian War.* New York: Harper & Brothers; 1836.
5. Geddes AM. The History of Smallpox. *Clinics in Dermatology.* 2006;24(3):152–157.
6. Papagrigorakis MJ, Yapijakis C, Synodinos PN, Baziotopoulou-Valavani E. DNA Examination of Ancient Dental Pulp Incriminates Typhoid Fever as a Probable Cause of the Plague of Athens. *International Journal of Infectious Diseases.* 2006;10(3):206–214.
7. Kazanjian P. Ebola in Antiquity? *Clinical Infectious Diseases.* 2015;61(6):963–968.
8. Cunha BA. The Cause of the Plague of Athens: Plague, Typhoid, Typhus, Smallpox, or Measles? *Infectious Disease Clinics of North America.* 2004;18(1):29–43.

9. Shapiro B, Rambaut A, Gilbert MTP. No Proof That Typhoid Caused the Plague of Athens (a Reply to Papagrigorakis et al.). *International Journal of Infectious Diseases.* 2006;10(4):334–335.

10. Ainley-Walker EW. General Pathology of Infection II. *The Clinical Journal.* 1902;21(Dec 31):169–175.

11. Crookshank EM. *History and Pathology of Vaccination.* Philadelphia: Blackiston; 1889.

12. Montagu MW. Town Ecologues: Saturday; The Small-Pox, Flavia. *Town Eclogues.* 1716. https://www.poetryfoundation.org/poems-and-poets/poems/detail/44766. Accessed October 20, 2016.

13. Paston G. *Lady Mary Wortley Montagu and Her Times.* London: Putnam's Sons; 1907.

14. Montagu MW. *Letters of the Right Honourable Lady M--y W-----y M------e: Written During Her Travels in Europe, Asia, and Africa, to Persons of Distinction, Men of Letters, &c. in Different Parts of Europe.* London: Cadell; 1784.

15. College of Physicians of Philadelphia. The History of Vaccines. 2017. http://www.historyofvaccines.org. Accessed February 27, 2017.

16. National Library of Medicine. Smallpox: A Great and Terrible Scourage. *History of Medicine.* 2002. https://www.nlm.nih.gov/exhibition/smallpox/sp_variolation.html. Accessed October 12, 2016.

17. Blakemore, E. How an African Slave in Boston Helped Save Generations from Smallpox. https://www.history.com/news/smallpox-vaccine-onesimus-slave-cotton-mather. Accessed July 25, 2019.

18. Boylston Z. *Historical Account of the Small Pox Inoculation in New England, Upon All Sorts of Persons, Whites, Blacks, and of All Ages and Constitutions.* London: Chandler; 1726.

19. Minardi M. The Boston Inoculation Controversy of 1721–1722: An Incident in the History of Race. *The William and Mary Quarterly.* 2004;61(1):47–76.

20. Ainley-Walker EW. *General Pathology of Inflammation, Infection, and Fever.* London: Lewis; 1904.

21. Riedel S. Edward Jenner and the History of Smallpox and Vaccination. *Proceedings (Baylor University Medical Center).* 2005;18(1):21–25.

22. Special Article on Immunity III. *Journal of the American Medical Association.* 1905;44(6):474–475.

23. Craigie D. *Elements of the Practice of Physic, Presenting a View of the Present State of Special Pathology and Therapeutics.* Edinburgh: Black; 1837.

24. Ogle W. Observations on Outbreaks of Diphtheria in Rural Districts. *St. George's Hospital Reports.* 1879;9(22):701–726.

25. Centers for Disease Control and Prevention. Diphtheria. *The Pink Book.* 2015. https://www.cdc.gov/vaccines/pubs/pinkbook/dip.html. Accessed March 2, 2017.

26. Jenner E. *An Inquiry into the Causes and Effects of the Variolae Vaccinae, a Disease Discovered in Some of the Western Counties of England, Particularly*

Gloucestershire and Known by the Name of Cow Pox. London: Sampson Low; 1798.

27. Creighton C. *Jenner and Vaccination: A Strange Chapter of Medical History.* Providence, RI: Snow & Farnham; 1892.

28. Simpson J, Weiner E. *Oxford English Dictionary.* Oxford, England: Oxford University Press; 1996.

29. Chantrey J, Meyer H, Baxby D, et al. Cowpox: Reservoir Hosts and Geographic Range. *Epidemiology and Infection.* 1999;122(3):455–460.

30. Shchelkunov SN, Safronov PF, Totmenin AV, et al. The Genomic Sequence Analysis of the Left and Right Species-Specific Terminal Region of a Cowpox Virus Strain Reveals Unique Sequences and a Cluster of Intact ORFs for Immunomodulatory and Host Range Proteins. *Virology.* 1998;243(2):432–460.

31. Qin L, Favis N, Famulski J, Evans DH. Evolution of and Evolutionary Relationships Between Extant Vaccinia Virus Strains. *Journal of Virology.* 2015;89(3):1809–1824.

32. Baxby D. The Origins of Vaccinia Virus. *The Journal of Infectious Diseases.* 1977;136(3):453–455.

33. Gubser C, Hué S, Kellam P, Smith GL. Poxvirus Genomes: A Phylogenetic Analysis. *Journal of General Virology.* 2004;85(1):105–117.

34. Weinstein RS. Should Remaining Stockpiles of Smallpox Virus (Variola) Be Destroyed? *Emerging Infectious Diseases.* 2011;17(4):681–683.

35. Director of Laboratory Science and Safety, FDA. FDA Review of the 2014 Discovery of Vials Labeled "Variola" and Other Vials Discovered in an FDA-Occupied Building on the NIH Campus. 2016, December 13. https://www.fda.gov/media/101811/download. Accessed April 18, 2019.

36. Fildes P. Richard Friedrich Johannes Pfeiffer. 1858–1945. *Biographical Memoirs of Fellows of the Royal Society.* 1956;2(Nov 1):237–247.

37. Metchnikoff É. *Immunity in Infective Diseases.* Cambridge, England: University Press; 1905.

38. Loos MM. Bacteria and Complement—A Historical Review. *Current Topics in Microbiology and Immunology.* 2013;121:1–5.

39. Buchner H. Immunitat, deren Naturliches Vorkommen und Kunstliche Erzeugung. *Münchener Medizinische Wochenschrift.* 1891;38(33):574–579.

40. Buchner H. Über die Nähere Natur der Bakterientötenden Substanz im Blutserum. *Zentralblatt Bakteriologie.* 1889;6(21):561–565.

41. Pfeiffer R. Weitere Mitteilungen über die Spezifischen Antikörper der Cholera. *Zeitschrift für Hygiene* 1894;18:1–16.

42. Ainley-Walker EW. General Pathology of Infection III. *The Clinical Journal.* 1903;21(Jan 14):202–208.

43. Wright AE, Douglas SR. An Experimental Investigation of the Role of the Blood Fluids in Connection with Phagocytosis. *Proceedings of the Royal Society of London.* 1903;72:357–370.

44. Wollstein M. An Immunologic Study of *Bacillus influenzae*. *Journal of Experimental Medicine*. 1915;22:445–456.

45. R. M. Martha Wollstein, M.D. 1868–1939. *American Journal of Diseases of Children*. 1939;58(6):1301.

46. Failure of Louis Wollstein and Company. *New York Times*. August 26, 1882, p. 8.

47. *The Trow (Formerly Wilson's) Copartnership and Corporation Directory of New York City*. New York: Trow; 1906.

48. Crawford PC. *Mill Supplies*. New York: Crawford; 1914.

49. *Polk's New York Copartnership and Corporation Directory: Boroughs of Brooklyn and Queens*. New York: Polk; 1915

50. Tebbe-Grossman J. Martha Wollstein. *The Encyclopedia of Jewish Women*. 2009. http://jwa.org/encyclopedia/article/wollstein-martha. Accessed December 29, 2015.

51. Wollstein M. Influenzal Meningitis and Its Experimental Production. *American Journal of Diseases of Children*. 1911;1(1):42–58.

52. Wollstein M. Serum Treatment of Influenzal Meningitis. *Journal of Experimental Medicine*. 1911;14(1):73–82.

53. von Behring E, Kitasato S. Uber das Zustandekommen Der Diphtherie-Immunitat Und der Tetanus-Immunitat Bei Thieren. In: Brock TD, ed. and trans., *Milestones in Microbiology: 1556 to 1940*. Washington, DC: ASM Press; 1890:138.

54. Wollstein M. Influenzal Meningitis: Experimental and Clinical. *Transactions of the Fifteenth International Congress of Hygiene and Demography, 1912*. 1913;2(Pt 1):57–62.

55. Mitchell LJ. *The Pathogenic Bacteria*. Philadelphia: Saunders; 1901.

56. Pfeiffer R, Kolle W. Weitere Untersuchungen über die spezifische Immunitatsreaktion der Cholera Vibrionen im Tierkörper und Reagensglase. *Zentralblatt fur Bakteriologie, Parasitenkunde und Infektionskrankheiten*. 1896;20(4):129–147.

57. Pfeiffer R, Kolle W. Experimentelle Untersuchungen zur Frage der Schutzimpfung des Menschen gegen Typhus absominalis. *Deutche Medizinische Wochenschrift*. 1896;22(2):735–737.

58. Noguchi H. The Thermostabile Anticomplementary Constituents of the Blood. *The Journal of Experimental Medicine*. 1906;8(6):726–753.

59. Wollstein M. Pfeiffer's Bacillus and Influenza: A Serological Study. *The Journal of Experimental Medicine*. 1919;30(6):555–568.

60. Wollstein M. The History of Women in Medicine. *The Woman's Medical Journal*. 1908;18(4):65–69.

61. Barry JM. *The Great Influenza: The Epic Story of the Deadliest Plague in History*. New York: Viking; 2004.

62. Jackson HC. Wollstein, Martha (1868–1939). *American National Biography Online*. 1999. https://www.anb.org/search?q=Wollstein&searchBtn=Search &isQuickSearch=true. Accessed March 6, 2017.

63. Abrams J, Wright, JR. Martha Wollstein: A Pioneer American Female Clinician-scientist. *Journal of Medical Biography*. 2018. https://doi.org/10.1177/0967772017743068.
64. Left Missing Sons $1 Each. *New York Times*, October 14, 1914.
65. Dr. Martha Wollstein. *New York Times*, October 1, 1939. https://timesmachine.nytimes.com/timesmachine/1939/10/01/94712493.html?pageNumber=55. Accessed July 26, 2019.

4

Finding the Capsule

BY 1928, THE SPANISH influenza pandemic had disappeared, the world had emerged from World War I, and families had long since buried their loved ones who had succumbed to the flu, the war, or both. Yet, the belief that the Spanish influenza, like the Russian influenza, had been caused by the bacterium *Bacillus influenzae* still lingered in the minds of many scientists. The newly proposed, alternative cause was a filterable agent—a novel kind of microbe that was found in the respiratory secretions of influenza patients. It was too tiny to see, even with a microscope. Its activity increased over time so it seemed to be alive. In laboratory experiments, patients' sputa, even after the specimens had been passed through a filter to remove bacteria, could transmit an influenza-like illness to rabbits and then from sick rabbits to well rabbits.[1] This filterable agent was a new notion, difficult to prove, and, at first, only reluctantly embraced by a few microbiologists. Later the "filterable agent" from patients with influenza disease would be identified as a virus, and its name would be influenza virus.

It was in 1928, while the argument about which microbe caused influenza still raged, that a motivated young woman named Margaret Pittman arrived at New York's Hospital of the Rockefeller Institute for Medical Research for postdoctoral training. As she considered her options, she recognized that "bacteriology was a relatively new and exciting biologic science"[2(p. 4)] and decided she wanted to study microbes. She was assigned to work in the Acute Respiratory Group, led

Continual Raving: A History of Meningitis and the People Who Conquered It. Janet R Gilsdorf, Oxford University Press (2020). © Oxford University Press.
DOI: 10.1093/oso/9780190677312.001.0001

by Dr. Oswald Avery, who handed her a timely research project: figure out if Pfeiffer's bacillus truly causes influenza.

Margaret Pittman was born in Prairie Grove, Arkansas, in 1901 (although her gravestone erroneously reads, "Jan. 20, 1902"[3]), the daughter of a "horse-and-buggy" country doctor, James Pittman, and his wife, Virginia, both descendants of early British immigrants. In their home "discipline, truth, love, and spiritual growth" nurtured young Margaret and her siblings, Helen and James, as they were introduced to the wonders of medicine. She seemed to have adored her father and described him as a passionate man who served all his patients "day or night, sunshine or rain. ... One time a cholecystectomy [surgical removal of the gallbladder] was performed, on a patient without funds, in a room of our house."[2(p. 3)] While still a schoolgirl, she administered anesthesia to a patient with a fractured leg while her father set the bone. She also assisted in vaccinating schoolchildren against smallpox.[2]

After high school, Margaret attended college in Siloam Springs, Arkansas, and studied music. She attributed "a spinal complication that has been a life companion" to her long hours of practicing the piano. The nature of that spinal problem remains unclear, but it resulted in discontinuation of her musical studies. She said she was not very talented, anyway.[2]

When Margaret was 18 years old, her father died suddenly from peritonitis following an appendectomy. She thought the infection might have been related to contaminated catgut suture used during the operation. On his deathbed, he instructed his wife that all their children must attend the Methodist college in Conway, Arkansas, so Margaret transferred to Hendrix College and majored in biology and mathematics. After her father's death, the family finances were severely depleted, so her mother sold home-canned fruits and vegetables and worked as a seamstress to support the children's education. There was no money for Margaret to pursue training as a physician. After college, she taught for 2 years at the Academy of Galloway Female College, and for 2 more years she worked on the Influenza Commission of the Metropolitan Life Insurance Company, where her job was to predict the impact of influenza on claims.[4] During those years, she squirreled away her money.

Margaret longed for some sort of work in the medical field, so she enrolled in the University of Chicago graduate school and paid for it from her savings and by babysitting at $0.35 an hour. The opportunities there were a good fit for her. In Margaret's words: "The spirit of research permeated the Department. As a student it was my high privilege to be associated with the scholarly faculty and the graduate students that were making outstanding contributions."[2](p. 4) Ultimately, she received a master's degree from the Department of Bacteriology and Hygiene under the mentorship of I. S. Falk; her master's thesis project was titled, "The S and R Colonial Forms of the Pneumococcus and Their Pathogenicity." She remained at the University of Chicago and was awarded a PhD under the mentorship of Mercy A. Southwith; her PhD thesis project was titled, "Pathogenesis of Experimental Pneumococcus Lobar Pneumonia."[2]

Pfeiffer's bacilli had baffled scientists since Richard Pfeiffer first discovered them. Their morphologic characteristics kept changing. When viewed under the microscope, the bacteria from culture plates sometimes appeared as cocci (tiny berries) or sometimes as bacilli (tiny ovals), and the oval shapes varied in their thickness so that they sometimes were fat like tiny chicken's eggs, other times skinny like grains of rice. Further, the bacteria in spinal fluid specimens were often elongated into threads. Sometimes, the thread-like forms absorbed Gram stain most intensely on their ends, sometimes not.[5] Thus, unlike other bacteria, they weren't uniform in appearance, which made their identification from clinical specimens difficult and interfered with understanding their nature and clinical implications. All strains, however, from either the meninges or the respiratory tracts of patients with meningitis, caused infection when injected into guinea pigs and mice, while only strains from the meninges were pathogenic in monkeys and rabbits.[6] The only consistent feature of the bacteria was their requirement for blood—horse, pigeon, human, or rabbit, but not sheep, blood—to grow. Someone needed to sort out all that confusion.

The first thing Pittman did on her arrival at the Rockefeller Institute was learn how to propagate *Hemophilus influenzae* in the laboratory. (Note: by the time Pittman published her work, *B. influenzae* had officially undergone a name change to *Hemophilus influenzae*, later

Haemophilus influenzae, because *bacillus*, meaning *rods*, wasn't specific enough, and *hemophilus* signified the bacteria's love of blood.) From her reading of the medical literature, she knew the *H. influenzae* bacillus, unlike the pneumococci from her prior work, wouldn't thrive on sheep blood agar, so she mixed molten nutrient agar with filtered, boiled horse blood, as had been described 6 years earlier by Levinthal and Fernbach.[7] With her research assistant, Salvatorus Spatolli, whom she described as her "able technician," Pittman poured the transparent Levinthal agar into petri plates, let the agar gel, and began to propagate the *H. influenzae* that had been collected from patients by her medical colleagues.[8] In all likelihood, it seemed very routine to her.

Several days later, she gazed at the shiny, little gray mounds on the agar, that is, the colonies of bacteria that were growing from a cerebrospinal fluid sample. They didn't all look alike. She studied them with the beam from her laboratory lamp cocked at an angle and aimed through the plate of clear agar from the back. Through the oblique light she saw two kinds of colonies growing from the one colony she had plated on the agar. In one variety, the colonies were opaque and goopy (she called them mucoid) and had an iridescent sheen. The others were smaller, had a faintly rough surface, and were more translucent. Pittman had discovered yet another difference among *H. influenzae*, and these characteristics were similar to the S and R pneumococcal colonies she had studied at the University of Chicago. So, she named the mucoid type of Pfeiffer's bacilli S for their smooth appearance and the other type R for rough (Figure 4.1). Bacteria from other patients with meningitis displayed the same two variations, Smooth and Rough, particularly those bacteria that had been repeatedly cultured in the laboratory over a number of months.[8]

Oswald Avery, Pittman's mentor at the Rockefeller, had identified the capsule (a structure made of strands of sugar that surrounded the bacteria like an overcoat) on the S (Smooth) pneumococci that was not present on R (Rough) strains. Thus, employing the gentian violet stain that Avery had used, Pittman looked for a capsule on the Smooth *H. influenzae* strains. When she examined the specimen under the microscope, she saw a faint sea-blue halo around many of the deeply purple-stained S bacteria, indicating that they also had a capsule. Further, the R colonies had no halo (Figure 4.2).[8] The presence of the

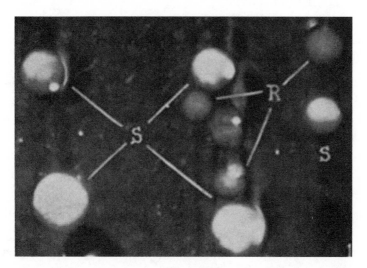

FIGURE 4.1 Photomicrograph of smooth (S) and rough (R) *H. influenzae* colonies growing on Levinthal agar as described by M. Pittman.

From Pittman M. Variation and Type Specificity in the Bacterial Species *H. influenzae*. *Journal of Experimental Medicine*. 1931;53:471–492. Courtesy of the *Journal of Experimental Medicine*.

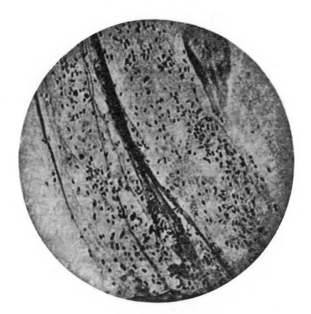

FIGURE 4.2 *Bacillus influenzae* in sputum. Halo around many of the bacteria represents the capsule.

From Hiss PH, Zinsser H. *A Text-book of Bacteriology, a Practical Treatise for Students and Practitioners of Medicine*. New York: Appleton; 1910:530.

capsule in some, but not all, strains explained at least some of the inconsistencies in Pfeiffer's bacilli that had confused so many scientists for so many years.

Pittman wanted to know if both the Smooth and the Rough strains caused infections, so she injected the bacteria into the abdomens or into the blood of mice, rats, and rabbits. She found that the Smooth strains were more pathogenic than the Rough strains; that is, compared to S strains, much higher doses of the R strains were needed to make the animals ill, and some R strains didn't sicken the animals at all, no matter how many bacteria she injected.[9] The discovery of the *Haemophilus* capsule promised to yield important new scientific paths for Pittman to follow, so she jettisoned her original research project—to prove whether *H. influenzae* caused influenza—and focused entirely on characterizing its capsule.

Previous investigators had shown immunologic differences between *H. influenzae* strains.[10–12] Was the capsule the reason for these immunological differences? Pittman wondered. To answer the question, she prepared antisera by immunizing a rabbit with a Smooth *H. influenzae* strain. When she tested the ability of the antisera to agglutinate several strains of the bacteria, she noted that the antisera gave a positive agglutination reaction with the Smooth but not the Rough strains, including a Rough strain that was a direct descendant of a Smooth strain after repeated subculturing. Pittman had read that Avery's pneumococcal capsule was water soluble, so she tested washings from Smooth *H. influenzae* strains and saw that they also reacted with the antisera. She concluded that, indeed, the immunologic differences among strains were related to the capsule.

Pittman asked herself if all *H. influenzae* capsules were immunologically alike. To answer that question, she collected capsulated strains from spinal fluids, blood, empyema fluid, throats of humans, and the nose of a monkey with tuberculosis. The *H. influenzae* strains are exclusively human bacteria and have never been isolated from native animals, so it's unclear what this last strain represented unless that laboratory monkey had been infected with *B. influenzae* in earlier experiments.

Pittman washed Smooth *H. influenzae* strains 35S, 41S, and 51S with water to obtain the water-soluble capsules and then immunized rabbits with each of the wash fluids. When she performed precipitation reactions using the resultant antisera, one strain, 35S, formed precipitates solely with its homologous serum (i.e., serum generated by immunization with strain 35S), while the other two strains failed to react with the 35S serum but reacted with each other's sera (Table 4.1).[9]

Thus, based on these immunologic reactions, Pittman had identified two distinct *H. influenzae* strains. She labeled the 35S strain "type a," and the 41S and 51S strains "type b." Among the fifteen strains with capsules she originally selected for her study, two were type a and thirteen were type b; of note, all seven meningitis strains were type b.

TABLE 4.1 Results of precipitation reactions, expressed as dilutions, when sera generated against three "Smooth" *H influenzae* strains (35S, 41S, and 51S) were tested with the three bacterial strains. The results show that when serum 35S [ie antibodies directed against strain 35S] is mixed with antigen [ie capsule] from strain 35 S, a strong precipitate results, shown by ++++, indicating that the antibodies have bound to the capsule. When serum 35S is mixed with either strain 41S or 51S, no precipitate forms, shown by -, indicating these two strains are immunologically different from strain 35S. Reactions of serum against strains 41S and 51S are similarly shown. The results of the experiment indicate that strains 41S and 51S are immunologically identical but both are different from strain 35S.

H. influenzae **precipitation reactions.**

Serum	Antigen	Final dilution of supernatant fluid							Controls
		1:2	1:4	1:8	1:16	1:32	1:64	1:128	
35S	35S	++++	++++	++++	++++	++++	++	+	—
"	41S	—	—	—	—				
"	51S	—	—	—	—				
41S	35S	—	—	—	—				
"	41S	++++	++++	++++	++++	++++	+++	+	—
"	51S	++++	++++	++++	++++	++++	+++	+	—
51S	35S								
"	41S	++++	++++	++++	++++	++++	+++	+	—
"	51S	++++	++++	++++	++++	++	++	+	—

From: Pittman, M. Variation and type specificity in the bacterial species *Hemophilus influenzae. Journal of Experimental Medicine.* 1931; 53:471–492. Courtesy of the *Journal of Experimental Medicine.*

Early in her work with the capsules of *H. influenzae*, Pittman noted that when she repeatedly passed the Smooth strains on agar plates, they often spawned a few Rough offspring, suggesting that during the passages, some of the Smooth bacteria had lost their capsules. She attempted the inverse experiment, looking for Smooth offspring from Rough strains. That, however, occurred only once, in a strain that had very recently converted to R from the S form. Thus, while S strains readily lost their capsules, it appeared extremely difficult for R strains to gain the ability to make the capsule. Many decades later, the genetic explanation for this phenomenon would be revealed: The size of the bacterial DNA that encodes the capsule is very large, too large for an R strain to acquire through gene exchange.[13,14] The single Rough → Smooth conversion Pittman witnessed probably represented several rare Smooth bacteria that had contaminated the Rough colony she had used.

Oswald Avery had shown that the capsules of pneumococci consisted of sugar molecules,[15] and Pittman assumed the same for *H. influenzae*. Walter Goebel, the chemist who worked on the pneumococci capsule with Avery, purified *H. influenzae* capsule for her. In her autobiography[2] and in her article describing horse antisera,[16] she mentioned, almost in passing, that she used Goebel's purified type b capsule in her precipitation reactions. In her article describing capsule serologic variation, she stated that Goebel was working on purifying type a capsules.[9] There is no record that the details of the purification procedures or the characterization of the purified capsule products were ever published, which is unusual, for most scientists eagerly share their results with other scientists and reap subsequent glory for their hard work. The likely explanation is that Goebel was too busy with his pneumococcal work and Pittman too busy actually using the isolated products in her experiments to spend time writing those papers.

Pittman continued to immunize many, many more rabbits with many, many Smooth *H. influenzae* and then tested the ability of the antisera from the rabbits to react with large numbers of strains. Ultimately, she identified six immunologically distinct types of Smooth *H. influenzae*, which she named types a through f.[17] The capsules, composed of complex sugar strands, are functionally more like nets than shells, in light of the fact that immune molecules as large as antibodies and complement (the protein in blood that enhances the ability of anti-bodies to kill bacteria) are able to attach to structures on the outer membrane of the bacteria beneath the capsule.

Pittman also didn't publish the data describing her discovery of types c through f capsules, but, rather, gladly shared with colleagues the antisera and the strains she had so meticulously characterized (which would be unheard of today). One of the recipients of her generosity was Dr. A. E. Platt, of the Government Laboratory of Bacteriology and Pathology in Adelaide, South Australia, who wrote, "In 1934, in a letter to the author [Platt], Miss [*sic*] Pittman stated that she had discovered other groups to the number of six which she designated a, b, c, d, e and f, and she kindly supplied me with cultures of type species of groups a, b, e and f, for which I now express my thanks."[18(p. 99)]

The Rough *H. influenzae* strains had no capsule when tested with the gentian violet stain, and when subjected to immunologic tests, they failed to react with the rabbit antisera prepared against capsule types a through f. These strains, which rarely cause meningitis, ultimately became known as "nontypeable" because, in lacking a capsule, they couldn't be typed with Pittman's antisera.

The quality of Pittman's work, and the diligence with which she pursued it, is evidenced by the fact that in the nearly 90 years since she identified the six capsule types, no additional types have been de-scribed. Thus, before she was 30 years old (Figure 4.3), Pittman had established the capsule, particularly the type b capsule, of *H. influenzae* as its primary virulence factor, and in the decades to come, the rest of the world would build on this observation to ultimately control the dis-eases, including meningitis, it causes. The type b capsule was the reason children got so sick with *H. influenzae* meningitis, the capsule was the focus of immune protection against this infection, and ultimately the capsule would become a vaccine to prevent such infections.

After 6 years as a research assistant, Pittman left the Rockefeller Institute in 1936 and worked as a bacteriologist at the New York State Department of Public Health for 2 years. In 1938, she followed her former University of Chicago Professor Sara Branham to the National Institutes of Health (NIH), where she worked until 1971, the year she met the required retirement age of 70 years.[19]

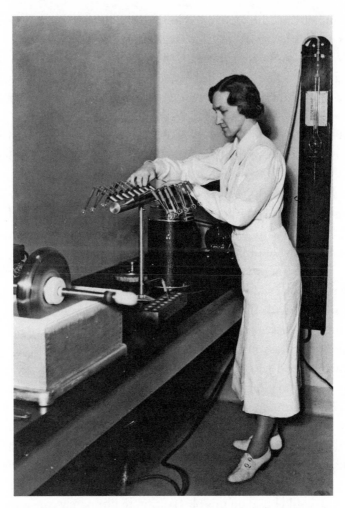

FIGURE 4.3 Dr. Margaret Pittman drying meningitis bacteria (circa 1937). Courtesy of the Office of History, National Institutes of Health. https://history.nih. gov/research/womenatnih.html.

At the NIH, she was instrumental in ensuring the safety, purity, and potency of all vaccines and therapeutic serums, toxins, and antitoxins used in the prevention, treatment, or cure of diseases or injuries, as mandated by the Congressional Biologics Control Act of 1902. Among many other accomplishments, she developed a potency assay for the pertussis vaccine, established methods to ensure the safety of blood products for soldiers in World War II, and standardized the cholera vaccine. In 1957 she was promoted to chief of the Laboratory of Bacterial Products, in the Division of Biologics Standards (Figure 4.4). She was the first woman named as chief of a major NIH laboratory and the first to be promoted to "supergrade GS-16".[2] Shortly after her retirement, the responsibilities of that division were transferred to the Food and Drug Administration (FDA), where they remain today.

I recently asked Dan Granoff, my long-standing friend and mentor, who introduced me to the wonders of *H. influenzae* many years ago, to share his recollections of Pittman. He had once published a paper with her.[20] Granoff wrote: "I recall writing a draft of the short manuscript and sending it to her for comments. She was 82 years old at the time and still active at the FDA. She returned the edited ms [manuscript] with handwritten comments (I wish I had saved it—darn). Her hand writing was impeccable (much like my Aunt Beatrice [Beatrice Trum Hunter, the prolific author of books on health and nutrition]) and her comments were like a school teacher, clear, concise, tactful and

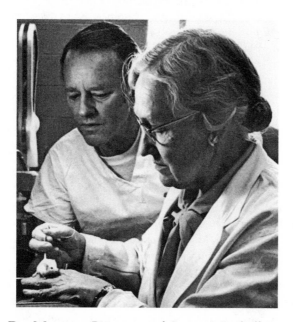

FIGURE 4.4 Dr. Margaret Pittman and James Marshall in 1971 at the National Institutes of Health, Division of Biologics.

From US Food and Drug Administration, Center for Biologics Evaluation and Research.

insightful. She also wrote to me that this paper would be her last on *H. influenzae*." (Granoff, personal communication).

Margaret Pittman was known as blunt, straight-to-the-point, systematic, and energetic. It was said that she "was always seeking and embracing the new, and could recognize new opportunities in new technologies."[21] As a retiree, she loved to garden; enjoyed traveling to faraway places, such as Cairo, Iran, Scotland, and Madrid, as a World Health Organization consultant[19]; and was active in the Mount Vernon United Methodist Church of Washington, DC. She died in Cheverly, Maryland, in 1995 at the age of 94 years and is buried in the Prairie Grove Cemetery in Arkansas. Etched into her gravestone are images of a microscope, a rack of test tubes, and the words, "A life devoted to the advancement of world health."[3]

References

1. Olitsky PK, Gates FL. Experimental Study of the Nasopharyngeal Secretions from Influenza Patients: Preliminary Report. *Journal of the American Medical Association.* 1920;74(22):1497–1499.
2. Pittman M. A Life With Biological Products. *Annual Review of Microbiology.* 1990;44(1):1–27.
3. Thiel T. My Famous File: Dr. Margaret Pittman. *Escape to the Silent Cities* (blog). 2010. http://escapetothesilentcities.blogspot.com/2010/05/my-famous-file-dr-margaret-pittman.html. Accessed October 12, 2016.
4. Ogilvie MB, Harvey JD. *The Biographical Dictionary of Women in Science: Pioneering Lives from Ancient Times to the Mid-20th Century.* New York: Routledge; 2000.
5. Ritchie J. On Meningitis Associated with an Influenza-like Bacillus. *The Journal of Pathology and Bacteriology.* 1910;14(4):615–627.
6. Wollstein M. Influenzal Meningitis and Its Experimental Production. *American Journal of Diseases of Children.* 1911;I(1):42–58.
7. Levinthal W, Fernbach H. Morphologische Studien an Influenzabacillen und das ätiologische Grippeproblem. *Zeitschrift für Hygiene und Infektionskrankheiten.* 1922;96(4):456–519.
8. Pittman M. The "S" and "R" Forms of *Hemophilus influenzae. Journal of Experimental Biology and Medicine.* 1930;27(4):299–301.
9. Pittman M. Variation and Type Specificity in the Bacterial Species *Hemophilus influenzae. The Journal of Experimental Medicine.* 1931;53(4):471–492.

10. Valentine E, Cooper GM. On the Existence of a Multiplicity of Races of *B. influenzae* as Determined by Agglutination and Agglutinin Absorption. *Journal of Immunology.* 1919;4(5):359–379.

11. Rivers TM, Kohn LA. The Biological and the Serological Reactions of Influenza Bacilli Producing Meningitis. *The Journal of Experimental Medicine.* 1921;34(5):477–494.

12. Povitzky OR, Denny HT, Provost DJ, LaMont AC. IV. Further Studies on Grouping of Influenza Bacilli with Special Reference to Permanence of Type in the Carrier. *The Journal of Immunology.* 1921;6(1):65–80.

13. Hoiseth SK, Gilsdorf JR. The Relationship Between Type b and Nontypable *Haemophilus influenzae* Isolated from the Same Patient. *The Journal of Infectious Diseases.* 1988;158(3):643–645.

14. Kroll JS. The Genetics of Encapsulation in *Haemophilus influenzae.* *The Journal of Infectious Diseases.* 1992;165:S93–S96.

15. Heidelberger M, Avery OT. The Soluble Specific Substance of Pneumococcus. *The Journal of Experimental Medicine.* 1923;38(1):73–79.

16. Pittman M. The Action of Type-Specific *Hemophilus influenzae* Antiserum. *The Journal of Experimental Medicine.* 1933;58(6):683–706.

17. Marrs CF, Krasan GP, McCrea KW, Clemans DL, Gilsdorf JR. *Haemophilus influenza*—Human Specific Bacteria. *Frontiers in Bioscience* 2001;6(September 1):e41–e60.

18. Platt AE. A Serological Study of *Haemophilus influenzae. Journal of Hygiene.* 1937;37(1):98–107.

19. National Library of Medicine. *Biographical Note: Margaret Pittman.* First published 2004; last updated May 17, 2019. https://oculus.nlm.nih.gov/ cgi/f/findaid/findaid-idx?c=nlmfindaid;idno=pittman590;view=reslist;di dno=pittman590;subview=standard;focusrgn=bioghist;cc=nlmfindaid;b yte=34248360. Accessed October 12, 2016.

20. Barenkamp SJ, Granoff DM, Pittman M. Outer Membrane Protein Subtypes and Biotypes of *Haemophilus influenzae* Type b: Relation Between Strains Isolated in 1934–1954 and 1977–1980. *Journal of Infectious Diseases.* 1983;148(6):1127.

21. Williams NA. Margaret Pittman (1901–1995). *Encyclopedia of Arkansas History & Culture* 2006. http://www.encyclopediaofarkansas.net/ encyclopedia/entry-detail.aspx?entryID=1738. Accessed October 12, 2016.

5

The Most Famous Graph in Microbiology

AFTER MARGARET PITTMAN DEMONSTRATED that *Haemophilus influenzae* possessed six distinct types of polysaccharide capsules, which she labeled a through f, and that patients with influenzal meningitis usually were infected with bacteria that carried the type b capsule, interest in this organism among pediatricians and scientists soared. Pittman's discovery opened new questions about *H. influenzae* and new doors for other scientists to further understand the infections it causes.

Joyce Wright, a pediatrician, and Hugh Ward, a physician/bacteriologist, at Harvard Medical School noted that a few individuals, mostly otherwise-healthy children, contracted *H. influenzae* type b meningitis, but most others didn't. Why was that? they wondered. To answer that question, they wanted to understand an important, but previously unstudied, aspect of meningitis: What was the relationship between virulence, or infection-causing capacity, of the bacteria and resistance (or susceptibility) of the host (i.e., a person or an animal) to the infection?

As much as Wright and Ward admired Pittman and her work, they didn't find her conclusion terribly convincing that *H. influenzae* possessing the type b capsule was more virulent than strains lacking a capsule.[1] In their opinion, Pittman showed that the number of Smooth (encapsulated) *H. influenzae* required to cause infections in rabbits was only slightly lower than that of Rough (nonencapsulated) *H. influenzae*, and this minor difference didn't seem all that significant. Based on earlier studies by Ward with *Streptococcus pneumoniae*,[2] they devised a better way to measure the virulence of *H. influenzae* strains. Rather

Continual Raving: A History of Meningitis and the People Who Conquered It. Janet R Gilsdorf, Oxford University Press (2020). © Oxford University Press. DOI: 10.1093/oso/9780190677312.001.0001

than the standard, laborious, and expensive standard technique of actually infecting rabbits with *H. influenzae* and measuring their survival, as Pittman had done, Wright and Ward assessed how well the bacteria in a test tube survived exposure to rabbit blood. Their idea was that bacteria *readily* killed by blood represented low-virulence organisms that wouldn't readily infect the animals, and those *rarely* killed by blood were high-virulence organisms capable of surviving in the bloodstreams of such hosts and thus causing infection.[3] In short, high-virulence bacteria were those poorly killed by blood and less likely to cause infection; conversely, low-virulence bacteria were those readily killed by blood and more likely to cause infection. In their assay, they mixed diluted rabbit blood with variable numbers of bacteria and assessed the ability of the bacteria to survive. They found that blood from healthy rabbits killed a million times more Rough *H. influenzae* strains than Smooth strains. These results confirmed what Pittman had found, that Rough (nonencapsulated) strains were less virulent (i.e., less able to survive in the rabbit's blood) than Smooth (encapsulated) strains.

Wright and Ward then used their killing assay to measure resistance or susceptibility of animals to infection.[3] In short, if blood from rabbit A killed *H. influenzae* better than blood from rabbit B, then rabbit A was more resistant, and rabbit B more susceptible, to infection with *H. influenzae*. In the course of their experiments, they confirmed Pfeiffer's phenomenon[4] that adding complement, the protein in serum than enhances antibody-mediated killing of bacteria, to the immune blood was key to facilitating bacterial killing (Figure 5.1),[5] such that

Immune blood + Bacteria + Complement → Dead bacteria

Further, Ward and Wright showed that immune whole blood worked as well as immune serum in the killing assays and could be used directly out of the animal without the tedious step of preparing serum from whole blood. They referred to this immune-mediated bacterial killing, which they correctly assumed represented antibody-mediated resistance to infection, as the "bactericidal power" of the blood.[5] In short, high killing power of an animal's blood (i.e., its bactericidal power)

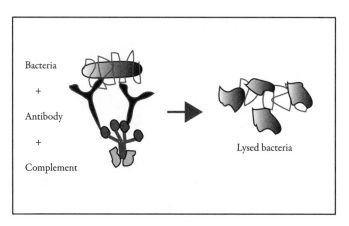

FIGURE 5.1 Bactericidal activity of antibodies and complement.
Drawing by the author.

against bacteria indicated high resistance of that animal to infection with those bacteria.

The word *bactericidal* represents an important concept in microbiology, with a colorful origin arising from contention. According to the *Oxford English Dictionary*,[6] the word, used as an adjective, simply means destructive to bacteria and first appeared during an argument between Charles Tyndall, an Irish physicist and polymath, and H. Charleston Bastian, an English physiologist and neurologist. Tyndall had been thinking about how organisms came into being and wrote a treatise on spontaneous generation, published in the magazine *The Nineteenth Century*. The treatise began as follows:

> WITHIN a ten minutes' walk of a little cottage which I have recently built in the Alps, there is a small lake, fed by the melted snows of the upper mountains. During the early weeks of summer no trace of life is to be discerned in this water; but invariably towards the end of July, or the beginning of August, swarms of tailed organisms are seen enjoying the sun's warmth along the shallow margins of the lake, and rushing with audible patter into the deeper water at the approach of danger. The origin of this periodic crowd of living things is by no means obvious.[7(p. 22)]

During the course of thinking about the beginnings of organisms, Tyndall wandered into the intellectual thicket of putrefaction and stated his support for the germ theory saying,

> Putrefaction begins as soon as bacteria, even in the smallest numbers, are admitted either accidentally or purposely. It progresses in direct proportion to the multiplication of the bacteria, it is retarded when they exhibit low vitality, and is stopped by all influences which either hinder their development or kill them. All *bactericidal* media are therefore antiseptic and disinfecting.[7(p. 22)]

Bastian took umbrage at Tyndall's essay and fired off a 16-page reply to *The Nineteenth Century* questioning Tyndall's theories of why organisms didn't grow in vessels that had been sterilized.[8] Bastian thought elevated physical pressure from the surrounding environment explained their failure to grow, while Tyndall thought it was because organisms hadn't been allowed to contaminate the sterile vessels. In his 11-page rebuttal to Bastian, Tyndall wrote the following:

> [In my original essay I stated that] animal and vegetable infusions had been subjected by me to mechanical pressures far more than sufficient to produce the bactericidal effects which his [Bastian's] theory ascribes to pressure, and that bacteria nevertheless grew and multiplied to countless swarms under such pressures."[8(p. 506)]

Thus, the word *bactericidal* was born.

As a young pediatrician at Boston Children's Hospital, Dr. Leroy Fothergill saw too many patients with bacterial meningitis. Distressed by both the seemingly large number of cases and their terrible outcomes, Fothergill and his colleague Dr. Lewis Sweet wondered what was causing those infections. They examined the medical records of meningitis patients between birth and 12 years old and found that over 40% of the cases were tuberculous meningitis, almost a quarter were meningococcal, while *H. influenzae*, pneumococcal, and hemolytic streptococcal meningitis were 10% each. What impressed Fothergill most was the young ages of the children with *H. influenzae* meningitis.

Further, in spite of the youthfulness of those patients, inexplicably very few newborns developed influenzal meningitis.[9]

Together with his colleague, the Harvard pediatrician Joyce Wright, Fothergill examined the relationship between the ages of the patients and the incidence of *H. influenzae* meningitis, using reports of the 200 cases described by Thomas Rivers[10] and by C. J. Bloom[11] in addition to his own 76 cases.[12] On a piece of graph paper, they plotted the numbers of cases on the vertical *y* axis and the ages of the patients on the longitudinal *x* axis. The resultant curve shot skyward at age 2 months, peaked between ages 6 and 9 months, and then slowly drifted downward until age 5 years, as depicted in Figure 5.2. After that, only rare, sporadic cases occurred.

Both Fothergill and Wright were curious and creative scientists, so they asked themselves, Why don't newborns get *H. influenzae* meningitis while slightly older children are dying from it with great regularity? And why do cases nearly disappear among older children? As they gazed at the graph, they developed a hypothesis: Newborns were protected against meningitis by immunity transferred by the blood of

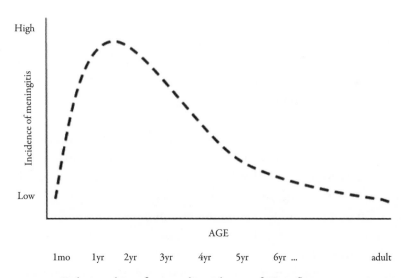

FIGURE 5.2 Relationship of age and incidence of *H. influenzae* meningitis. Drawing by the author with data from Fothergill LD, Wright J. Influenzal Meningitis: The Relation of Age Incidence to the Bactericidal Power of Blood Against the Causal Organism. *Journal of Immunology.* 1933;24:273–284.

their immune mothers, through their placentas, to the babies. Further, the maternal immunity bestowed on the newborns was short-lived as it seemed to disappear by 2 to 3 months of age, at which time the babies became more susceptible to *H. influenzae* infection. Then, after 2 years of age, infection dropped off because, they surmised, the children began to develop natural immunity that would protect them for the rest of their lives.

They proceeded to try to prove that hypothesis by building on the previous study of Ward and Wright,[5] who showed that the inability of normal rabbit blood to kill *H. influenzae* was a good measure of the bacteria's virulence; the more vigorously blood killed the bacteria, the less virulent was the bacteria. Fothergill and Wright declared the following:

> The invasion of an animal by a living organism is determined by the relation between the resistance of the animal and the virulence of the organism. It was considered, therefore, that when, as in this case, the virulence of the organism is known to be constant, the resistance of an individual may be measured indirectly by the bactericidal power of the blood.[12(p. 276)]

Thus, they employed the bactericidal assay to prove their hypothesis. They mixed blood from 133 children with various dilutions of Smooth *B. influenzae* (they still used the old name *Bacillus influenzae*) from a patient with meningitis and incubated the mixtures for 18 hours. They then removed a wire loopful of the bacteria-blood mixture from each tube and cultured it on chocolate agar. The blood from newborns killed a large number of bacteria, blood from children 2–3 months to 2 years killed none to few, and blood from children older than 5 years killed large numbers. Therefore, they had proven their hypothesis: The power of blood to kill *B. influenzae* was highest in blood from newborns and from children over years old, while the blood of children between those ages had little killing power, as reflected in Figure 5.3.

Fothergill and Wright then superimposed the two graphs—the number of cases and the bactericidal titers of the blood of healthy children by age—and the legendary Fothergill and Wright graph came alive. The new image showed the beautiful dynamic of immunity

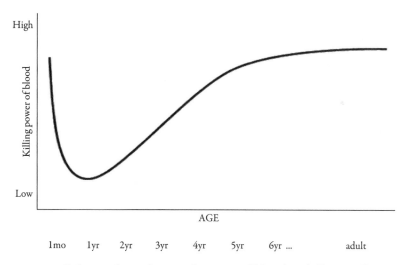

FIGURE 5.3 Relationship of age and power of blood to kill *H. influenzae.* Drawing by the author with data from Fothergill LD, Wright J. Influenzal Meningitis: The Relation of Age Incidence to the Bactericidal Power of Blood Against the Causal Organism. *Journal of Immunology.* 1933;24:273–284.

in two graceful arching lines that intersected in two places, at ages 2 months and 3 years (Figure 5.4). Like a dance, the ebbs and flows in the incidence of *B. influenzae* meningitis after birth changed with the changing bactericidal activity of the children's blood as they aged.[12] It is likely the most famous graph in all of bacteriology, taught in nearly every microbiology/immunology class in the world, a memorable way to understand the unique epidemiology of bacterial meningitis in children. More important, the graph represents a paradigm shift in the understanding of meningitis: Susceptibility to the infection is inversely related to the power of the blood to kill the bacteria (e.g., immunity and both susceptibility and immunity are related to age).

Further, the graph demonstrates that newborn babies are protected against *B. influenzae* infection by the high level of the killing power in their blood, and Fothergill and Wright had correctly surmised that protection was due to antibodies that had been passed through the placenta from a mother's blood to her unborn baby. Then, shortly after birth, the antibodies are degraded in the baby and immunity disappears. While this study of maternally derived passive immunity in

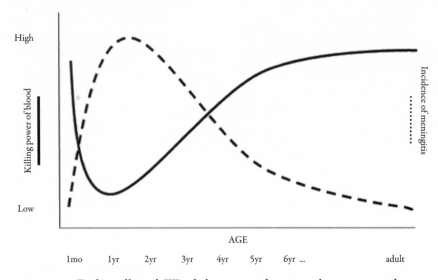

FIGURE 5.4 Fothergill and Wright's curves showing the inverse relationship of incidence of *H. influenzae* meningitis and power of blood to kill *H. influenzae* by age.

Drawing by the author with data from Fothergill LD, Wright J. Influenzal Meningitis: The Relation of Age Incidence to the Bactericidal Power of Blood Against the Causal Organism. *Journal of Immunology.* 1933;24:273–284.

babies was not a new observation—Paul Ehrlich and Louis Vaillard had observed that newborn rabbit and guinea pig pups of mothers immunized with tetanus or anthrax, respectively, were protected against these infections, and the protection had disappeared by the time the pups were 3 months old[13]—it was early scientific documentation of maternally derived, passive immunity related to a human infection. The basic principle of transplacentally acquired, but short-lived, protection against the common causes of meningitis in children has also been demonstrated for meningococci[14] and for pneumococci.[15]

While Joyce Wright was a key investigator in these important scientific studies, time has unfortunately erased many details of her life. According to a review of women who worked with *H. influenzae*, she was born in 1903 or 1904[16]; based on European birth records, she was likely born December 8, 1903, in Chorley, Lancashire, England.[17] A list of medical school graduates published in the *British Medical Journal* documented that she received her medical training at the University of Oxford in the United Kingdom, and in 1926 she earned her BM, BCh (British degrees equivalent to MD, for medical doctor, in the United States).[18] In the early 1930s, she was a research fellow in bacteriology at Harvard Medical School, where she worked with Ward and Fothergill on immunity against *H. influenzae*. In 1936, while working as a bacteriologist in Capetown, South Africa, she received a research fellowship from the British Medical Research Council to study the bacteria that cause diphtheria.[19] This fellowship award was granted to "encourage young British medical graduates of special ability and original mind towards becoming investigators in those branches of medical science which are concerned directly with disease as it occurs in human beings."[20(p. 1212)] By 1940, she had moved to London, where she worked for many years as a staff member of the Medical Research Council and published a number of papers related to bacteriology and epidemiology, using the advanced degree title she had subsequently been awarded: Joyce Wright, DM. She died in 1991 in Chelmsford, Essex, England.[16,17]

Leroy Dryden Fothergill was born in Carson City, Nevada, on April 15, 1901, the eldest of Theodore and Clara (née Peterson) Fothergill's six children.[21] After graduating from the University of Nevada, he worked at a university agricultural experiment station for a year before enrolling in medical school at Harvard University. He graduated in 1929, cum laude, and worked at Children's Hospital in Boston for a number of years as a consultant in infectious diseases and director of the bacteriology laboratory. After leaving Boston, he served as a naval officer, conducting epidemiologic investigations of infectious diseases, and, later in his life, became associate director of the Center for Zoonoses Research at the University of Illinois.[22]

As an expression of his strong interest in the ecologic and social consequences of infectious diseases, Fothergill served as a scientific advisor to the Chemical Corps, which focused on biologic warfare projects at Fort Detrick, Maryland, home to the US biological defense program (Figure 5.5). He was committed to defense against biologic weapons, stating, "Since any enemy nation might be expected to use all the weapons in its arsenal, it would follow that it would give serious consideration to biological warfare. Because of this possibility it is incumbent upon each of us to become fully acquainted with the nature

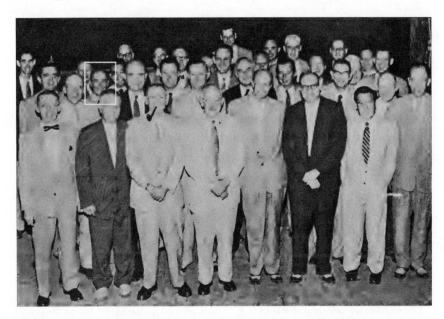

FIGURE 5.5 Fort Detrick Chemical Corps Advisory Counci!, October 5, 1954. Dr. Leroy Fothergill, boxed.

From Covert NM. Cutting Edge: A History of Fort Detrick, Maryland 1943–1993. US Army Garrison, Fort Detrick, MD: Public Affairs Office; 1993.

of biological warfare."[23(p. 865)] He recognized the value of applying the knowledge of infectious agents and the diseases they cause, as well as the principles of public health, to building both community and military programs to defend against attacks with microbial weapons. He was very serious about excellence in the conduct of science and received a commendation from his superiors at Fort Detrick for his insistence that scientific procedures be rigidly followed.[24]

While at Fort Detrick, back when it was in the business of developing biological weapons, Fothergill reportedly gave a tour of the facility to Matthew Meselson, a geneticist and molecular biologist with an interest in biologic warfare. As they walked through the building that housed the giant, whirring, stainless steel fermenters and separators used to purify the toxin of *Bacillus anthracis* (the agent of anthrax), Meselson asked, "Why do we do this?"

Fothergill replied, "It's a lot cheaper than nuclear weapons."[25(p. 42)]

He had correctly interpreted the question as "why America was doing this?" His own work involved defensive strategies against biologic warfare, not in developing offensive weapons. His papers are heavy on the details of microbial aerosol trajectories under various weather conditions; the threats of exotic infectious agents such as those that cause Q fever, Rift Valley fever, and louping-ill in sheep; and lethal doses of specific pathogens.[26] Yet, Fothergill strongly believed in science as a moral agent, and that scientists had the responsibility of carrying that morality forward through their work.

References

1. Pittman M. Variation and Type Specificity in the Bacterial Species *Hemophilus influenzae*. *The Journal of Experimental Medicine*. 1931;53(4):471–492.

2. Ward HK. Observations on the Phagocytosis of the Pneumococcus by Human Whole Blood: I. The Normal Phagocytic Titre, and the Anti-Phagocytic Effect of the Specific Soluble Substance. *The Journal of Experimental Medicine*. 1930;51(5):675–684.

3. Wright J, Ward HK. Studies on Influenzal Meningitis II. B. Influenzae— The Problem of Virulence and Resistance. *The Journal of Experimental Medicine*. 1932;55(2):235–246.

4. Pfeiffer R. Weitere Mitteilungen über die spezifischen Antikörper der Cholera. *Zeitschrift für Hygiene*. 1894;18:1–16.

5. Ward HK, Wright J. Studies on Influenzal Meningitis I. The Problems of Specific Therapy. *The Journal of Experimental Medicine*. 1932;55(2):223–234.

6. Simpson J, Weiner E. *Oxford English Dictionary*. Oxford, England: Oxford University Press; 1996.

7. Tyndall J. Spontaneous Generation. *The Nineteenth Century*. 1878;3(11):22–47.

8. Bastian HC. Spontaneous Generation: A Reply. *The Nineteenth Century*. 1878;3(12):261–277.

9. Fothergill LD, Sweet LK. Meningitis in Infants and Children with Special Reference to Age-Incidence and Bacteriologic Diagnosis. *The Journal of Pediatrics*. 1933;2(6):696–710.

10. Rivers TM. Influenzal Meningitis. *American Journal of Diseases of Children*. 1922;24(2):102–124.

11. Bloom CJ. Influenzal Meningitis is Amenable to Treatment. *New Orleans Medical and Surgical Journal*. 1931(7);83:455–466.

12. Fothergill LD, Wright J. Influenzal Meningitis: The Relation of Age Incidence to the Bactericidal Power of Blood Against the Causal Organism. *Journal of Immunology*. 1933;24(4):273–284.

13. The Heredity of Acquired Immunity. *Journal of Comparative Pathology and Therapeutics.* 1888;9:71–77.

14. Goldschneider I, Gotschlich EC, Artenstein MS. Human Immunity to the Meningococcus. *Journal of Experimental Medicine.* 1969;129(6):1307–1326.

15. Sutliff WD, Finland M. Antipneumococcic Immunity Reactions in Individuals of Different Ages. *The Journal of Experimental Medicine.* 1932;55(6):837–852.

16. O'Brien KL, Anderson PW. Leaning In to the Power of the Possible: The Crucial Role of Women Scientists on Preventing *Haemophilus influenzae* Type b Disease. *Pediatric Infectious Diseases Journal.* 2014;33(3):280–283.

17. Family Search. *Joyce Wright.* https://familysearch.org/search/record/results?count=20&query=%2Bgivenname%3AJoyce~%20%2Bsurname%3AWright~%20%2Bbirth_place%3AEngland~%20%2Bbirth_year%3A1903-1904. Accessed July 29, 2017.

18. Universities and Colleges: University of Oxford. *British Medical Journal.* 1926;2(3419):137.

19. Wright J. Types of *C. diphtheriae* in Capetown. *British Medical Journal.* 1937;1(3970):259–260.

20. Studentships and Research Fellowships. *British Medical Journal.* 1936;2(3962):1212.

21. Family Search. Leroy Fothergill. https://familysearch.org/search/record/results?count=20&query=%2Bgivenname%3ALeroy~%20%2Bsurname%3AFothergill~%20%2Bbirth_place%3A%22Carson%20City%20Nevada%22~. Accessed July 29, 2017.

22. Glassman HN. Leroy Dryden Fothergill, 1901–1967. *New England Journal of Medicine.* 1968;278(18):1025.

23. Fothergill LD. Biological Warfare and Its Defense. *Public Health Reports (1896–1970).* 1957;72(10):865–871.

24. Covert NM. *Cutting Edge: A History of Fort Detrick Maryland, 1943–1993.* Fort Detrick, Maryland: Public Affairs Office, Headquarters US Army Garrison; 1993.

25. Klotz LC, Sylvester EJ. *Breeding Bio Insecurity: How US Biodefense is Exporting Fear, Globalizing Risk, and Making Us All Less Secure.* Chicago: University of Chicago Press; 2009.

26. Fothergill LD. The Biological Warfare Threat. In: Staff of the American Chemical Society, ed. *Nonmilitary Defense* (Vol. 26). Washington, DC: American Chemical Society; 1960:23–33.

6

Early Treatment—Immune Serum from a Horse

IT WAS DEEP IN winter at the dawn of 1893, a notably severe January with heavy falls of snow and frigid temperatures alternating with short thaws, that epidemic meningitis broke out among Cumberland coal miners. The cases apparently started at a dance shortly after the new year. It was a "bitterly cold night and ... two young men overheated themselves and subsequently became severely chilled; both developed the disease the next day."[1(p.70)] Subsequently, more and more cases emerged, and they were said to be often associated with cold snaps. In reality, the chill didn't directly cause their illnesses, although the stress of being cold may have increased their susceptibility to the infection.

The governor of Maryland sent an urgent request to Johns Hopkins Medical School for someone to investigate the outbreak. A young professor of pathology, Dr. Simon Flexner, and his associate, Llewellys Barker, were assigned to determine the cause of the new epidemic.

On first blush, the initial town they encountered, Lonaconing, population about 5,000, sounded idyllic:

> The town is situated in a narrow valley and extends well up the sides of the steep hills which enclose it. Through the bottom of the gulch runs a muddy stream known as George's Creek. The mountains rise more or less abruptly from the edges of the creek. ... The stream and valley are somewhat tortuous at this spot, and give the place the appearance of being surrounded on all sides by mountains.[2(p. 156)]

Continual Raving: A History of Meningitis and the People Who Conquered It. Janet R Gilsdorf, Oxford University Press (2020). © Oxford University Press.
DOI: 10.1093/oso/9780190677312.001.0001

When Flexner and Barker dug deeper into the outbreak, however, things appeared pretty grim in the four Appalachian towns involved in the epidemic: Lonaconing, Frostburg, Ocean, and Barton. "Sanitary conditions were about as unhygienic as could be well imagined," they wrote in their preliminary report.

> In Lonaconing ... a river [George's Creek] runs through the center of the town and acts as a main sewer. The houses in the town were for the most part built in rows, tier above tier upon the sides of the steep hills which rise from either band of the creek. The outhouses belonging to the dwellings were placed flat upon the ground and usually upon a higher plane. During a thaw or rainstorm, the sewage and refuse from the upper yards, outhouses, and stables were washed down through the premises and past the dwellings of those who lived below. Upon the margins of the creek, in the very center of the town, were located the slaughter-houses, and refuse from these found its way unforbidden into the stream. The water supply of the place was derived chiefly from wells, and these were frequently contaminated with surface washings.[1(p. 169)]

Up to that time, most investigators considered epidemic meningitis to have a miasmic origin (related to "bad air") rather than a bacterial origin. During the autopsies that Flexner and Barker conducted on patients who died of meningitis, however, they found the infecting bacteria in the brain as well as in the nasal passages, leading them to conclude that the central nervous system disease was the result of bacterial contamination from the respiratory system. They didn't propose a potential mechanism for that to occur, however, and offered no speculation regarding how the bacteria traveled from the nose to the brain. In addition, because of the appalling conditions of the households in Lonaconing, they concluded that the illness represented "a predisposition of the whole community outside the merely personal predisposition."[2(p. 273)] Thus, they felt that, in addition to bacteria causing the infection (rather than bad air), both individual (patient) risk factors such as inadequate hygiene and exposure to cold and environmental risk factors such as poor sanitation contributed to the infection. Ultimately, scientists have learned that Flexner was right about the bacteria but not about poor hygiene and sanitation as playing roles in developing meningitis. Medical scientists now also know that cold weather has little to do with it.

Flexner and Barker called the bacteria they saw on smears and grew on cultures of the spinal fluid from a patient at Lonaconing *Micrococcus lanceolatus*.[2] The name reflects what they saw under the microscope: small, round (thus the term *micrococcus*) bacteria that were, on closer scrutiny, lancet shaped. Later, Anton Weichselbaum would call these bacteria *Diplococcus intracellularis*, reflecting that the round (coccus) bacteria are found in pairs (diplo) and inside white blood cells (intracellularis)[3]; they are now called *Neisseria meningitidis* to honor Dr. Albert Neisser, who discovered their cousin, *Neisseria gonorrheae*, the cause of gonorrhea.[4,5]

Suddenly in May 1893, the meningitis outbreak in the Appalachian coal-mining towns ended abruptly (as they always did, for unknown reasons). Over 200 cases were identified during the previous 5 months. Forty percent of the patients died.[1] Flexner returned to Baltimore with the new understanding that, because "all classes suffered the infection—strong and weak, well-to-do and poor"—epidemic meningitis resulted from a predisposition of the entire community to the infection rather than merely a predisposition of the individuals.

Simon Flexner was born in 1863, in Louisville, Kentucky, the fourth of nine children (Figure 6.1). His mother, Esther Abraham, a dressmaker prior to her marriage, hailed from Alsace and emigrated from Paris to the United States. His father, Morris Flexner, emigrated from Bohemia, survived yellow fever in Louisiana, worked his way up the Mississippi and Ohio Rivers, and settled in Kentucky, where he became, first, a peddler and then a hat merchant.[6]

As a shy and timid boy in a crowded, rowdy household, Simon became a reader. Yet, he detested school and described it as a "dreary, uninteresting place." To entertain himself, he engaged in mischief. His punishment at the hands of a teacher named Miss Johnston included daily lashes with a strap. Simon's lackadaisical attitude about school earned him the most dreaded of sentences—he had to repeat the fifth grade.[7]

Simon was also a dreamer. In spite of being "small in stature and weak in muscle," underappreciated by his teammates, and exiled to the

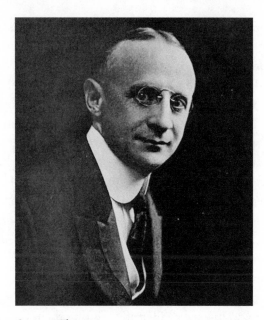

FIGURE 6.1 Dr. Simon Flexner.

From picture of Simon Flexner.jpg. Photographed by Elias Goldensky. US public domain photo.https://commons.wikimedia.org/wiki/File:Picture_of_Simon_Flexner.jpg.

outfield where the baseballs never landed, he enjoyed playing "town ball" in the streets of Louisville. Standing alone far behind third base in the shadows of the surrounding buildings, he imagined himself as a star baseball player, a hero who saved the day in close games. For the rest of his life, Simon treasured those vivid childhood visions of grand success.

When he was in sixth grade, Simon decided he had had enough of school and didn't return after the Christmas holidays. In fact, he never went back at all—didn't finish elementary school, didn't attend high school or college. Rather, he bounced from lowly odd job to even lowlier odd job until he suffered "a brush with death" from typhoid fever, which "ignited in him an intellectual purpose."[8] Following in the footsteps of his oldest brother, Jacob, Flexner apprenticed in a drug store and became a pharmacist.

While working as a druggist, he decided to give the medical school in Louisville a try. The coursework at the medical school consisted of 4 months of lectures, repeated again in the second year.[6] The only laboratory course was dissection, and the bacteriology course consisted of readings from T. M. Prudden's *Story of the Bacteria*, where he learned (erroneously) that bacteria were plants, related to algae.[9] Such was the archaic nature of medical education at that time. After 2 years of medical studies, he graduated in 1889, the year of the Russian influenza pandemic. Following graduation, Simon didn't serve an 8-month apprenticeship, as was customary but not mandatory, and he never applied for a license to practice medicine. Rather, he found his way to Baltimore, where he pestered the eminent Dr. William Henry Welch at Johns Hopkins University into allowing him to study pathology in his laboratory. Ultimately, Simon became a professor at the newly established Johns Hopkins Medical School.

In the late 1800s, at the time Flexner attended medical school, the education of physicians was a haphazard affair. Many schools that trained physicians were commercial ventures run by practicing doctors whose major objective was profit making rather than sound medical training. Students were lured to these schools by brochures filled with exaggeration, misstatements, and half-truths that portrayed medicine as a business rather than a profession.[10] Not uncommonly, their advertising budgets exceeded the medical studies budgets. The result was an oversupply of poorly trained physicians.

In 1910, the Carnegie Foundation funded an examination of the status of medical education in the United States and Canada and recruited Simon Flexner's older brother Dr. Abraham Flexner to conduct it. Abraham was an educator, not a physician, and during his visits to each American medical school, he found a lot to criticize. The Flexner Report, as it is called, described three types of medical schools: (1) "those that require two or more years of college work for entrance"; (2) "those that demand actual graduation from a four-year high school or oscillate about its supposed 'equivalent'"; and (3) "those that ask little more than the rudiments or the recollection of a common school education." [10(p. 28)] The medical school in Louisville that Simon Flexner attended was of the third type.

At the time Abraham Flexner visited the University of Louisville Medical Department in Louisville, approximately 20 years after his brother Simon had graduated, the entrance requirement was less than a high school education. Six hundred students were enrolled. The teaching hospital had 50 beds, with an average of 30 patients. Abraham Flexner judged the hospital facilities to be poor in respect to both quality and extent.[10]

The Flexner Report led to major reforms in medical education. Many substandard medical schools closed, and those that survived became associated with institutions of higher education, with full-time faculty and curricula based on the basic medical sciences of anatomy, physiology, pathology, and pharmacology. Two years of college preparation, including courses in chemistry, physics, and biology, were required for enrollment.

In late 1904, epidemic meningitis struck again, this time in New York City's Lower East Side during a hard winter of bone-rattling cold and thigh-high snow. Immigrant families, particularly the Italians and Russians, suffered most from the scourge that raced through the teeming tenements.[11] In the words of the muckraking, three-time Pulitzer Prize–winning journalist[12] Burton Hendrick in *McClure's Magazine*,

> A child would go to bed apparently well and happy, and, before sunlight, begin tossing in the advanced stages of the disease. Children suddenly fell unconscious at play, and became acutely ill before they could be put to bed. [Those afflicted had head pain] as if nails and screws were forced into the brain. Frequently, the wildest delirium supervenes: the child shrieks and tosses so convulsively upon the bed that the strength of grown men is sometimes needed to hold it down. ... Sometimes the impact of simple sunlight upon the skin produces convulsions; quickly closing or shutting a door precipitates a spasm, and moving the child even slightly upon its bed is absolute torture. At other times the victim lies comatose and paralyzed; a heavy anesthesia settles upon the body; one can rub a cotton swab roughly over the eyeball without producing the slightest sensation.[13(p. 594)]

Such was the 1904–1905 outbreak of epidemic cerebrospinal meningitis in New York City, the worst ever reported in the United States up to that time. In greater New York, 3,799 people contracted the disease and 2,594 died, for a fatality rate of 70%.[11] Two-thirds of its victims were children under 10 years of age; girls and boys were equally afflicted. Cases appeared in clusters, affecting groups of people at about the same time and in the same geographic region. Death came most commonly to the very young and to those in middle and older ages.[14]

Mortality from epidemic meningitis could be swift or lingering and followed one of three patterns: (1) the few with fulminant disease who died within 6 to 36 hours of becoming ill; (2) the majority, whose symptoms gradually intensified over 6 to 10 days and terminated in death; and (3) the few whose symptoms stabilized to a chronic state that lasted for weeks or months until they died.[14]

Survivors were infrequent. Among those, the disease resolved either by lysis (a gradual decline of the symptoms) or by crisis. In the more common form, by lysis, the acute symptoms gradually improved until recovery was achieved, often over weeks or months. In the uncommon form, by crisis, the acute symptoms abruptly, inexplicably resolved several days after they began.

As Hendrick further wrote,

Dark purplish spots break out all over the body, and small ulcerous swellings disfigure the lips and face. The patient lies with the knees drawn up and the muscles rigid and contracted, as in lockjaw; the head and neck turn backward, and sometimes the spine, as in the latter disease, almost doubles upon itself [Figure 6.2]. If the disease is protracted, a frightful emaciation takes place and the child frequently becoming [sic] little more than a breathing skeleton.[13(p. 595)]

Hendrick went on to describe the paucity of those with complete recovery; the survivors, instead, were often left blind, deaf, or sometimes both. Some were permanently paralyzed, and others developed hugely swollen heads, indicative of hydrocephalus ("water on the brain"). "In some instances, the meningitis germ had attacked children [sic] bright, happy and physically robust and left them incurable imbeciles."[13(p. 596)] And yet, a surprising number of survivors were intellectually normal irrespective of the gravity of their illness.[14]

Nevertheless, the disease was so feared, its symptoms so horrible, and its outcome so dismal that the Health Department of New York City established a special commission to investigate the meningitis

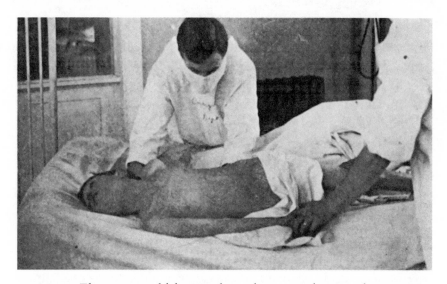

FIGURE 6.2 Eleven-year-old boy with epidemic cerebrospinal meningitis with opisthotonos (arched back).

From Sophian A. *Epidemic Cerebrospinal Meningitis.* St. Louis, MO: Mosby; 1913:73.

epidemic. The commission was divided into two sections, one responsible for conducting studies of the clinical manifestations of the illness and the other for conducting studies of the bacteria isolated from the patients. Simon Flexner, by then the director of the newly established Rockefeller Institute of Medical Research, was appointed to the bacteriology section of the commission.[13]

Primed by his experience with epidemic meningitis in Maryland coal miners, Flexner, in his role as a member of the Health Department Commission, set to work on the New York meningitis epidemic in the winter of 1904 and spring of 1905. He confirmed that it also was caused by *D. intracellularis* (also known as meningococci), although he was able to isolate the bacteria from only a few of the New York patients and relied on local physicians, including Dr. Martha Wollstein at Babies' Hospital in New York City (who studied immunity against *Haemophilus influenzae*), to provide him with additional bacterial isolates. He had difficulty growing the bacteria in his laboratory. Finally, following a suggestion from a Dr. W. H. Park of the Health Department, he landed on a magic concoction for the culture medium: diluted sheep serum mixed with beef broth, glucose, and agar-agar.[15]

But, to his frustration, when Flexner finally coaxed the bacteria to grow on the agar, they quickly disappeared, a phenomenon now recognized as spontaneous autolysis. The irony was huge: Bacteria that were robust enough to cause such terrible infections in people enigmatically self-destructed after 2 or 3 days while growing in the laboratory. Thus, Flexner needed to reculture the bacteria on fresh agar plates every 1 or 2 days to sustain live bacteria for his experiments on the pathogenic properties of *D. intracellularis*.

During each of the 2 years of the New York epidemic, 10 times as many people were infected as during any of the previous 37 years.[11] It spontaneously subsided in 1905, after approximately 4,000 people had been infected and 3,429 died. Flexner calculated the mortality rate to be 73.5%.[15]

Beyond being trained as a physician (sort of), Flexner was an extremely curious man and an intellectual who yearned to understand meningitis better. Why were some strains more pathogenic than others? What about those strains made them pathogenic at all? Toward that end, consistent with the standard for studying most other infections at that time, he tried to establish meningitis in animals by infecting them with meningococci isolated from patients in the New York epidemic. Mice seemed resistant to the bacteria, guinea pigs varied in their susceptibility, and finally, he successfully established meningeal infection in monkeys by injecting bacteria directly into the animals' spinal columns.[16,17] When he examined the pathologic specimens from the infected monkeys under the microscope, the tissues of the inflamed brains looked exactly like those of children who had died of meningitis (Figure 6.3).

Flexner used different strains of the bacteria to infect each monkey, strains named for the children they had originally infected: Kepp, Bingly, Goldman, Cohn, Smith, Behren, Whitaker, and Gratz. This practice is absolutely prohibited today out of respect for the patients and for the HIPAA (Health Insurance Portability and Accountability Act of 1996) law, which forbids public identification of patients without their permission. Since the 1980s, bacterial strains are designated by numbers or letters that may indicate the name of an investigator or the body site/ geographic location from which the microbes were isolated. Occasionally,

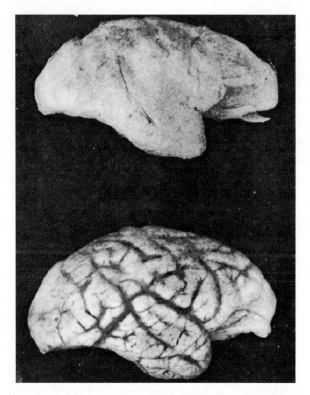

FIGURE 6.3 Brains of two monkeys with experimental meningitis. Top, the monkey had chronic meningitis with exudate covering the entire surface so that the natural gyrations of the brain cannot be seen. Bottom, the monkey had acute meningitis; the blood vessels of the meninges are dilated and clearly seen.

From Flexner S. Experimental Cerebrospinal Meningitis in Monkeys. *Journal of Experimental Medicine.* 1907;9:142–167.

however, classic, heirloom strains are still called by their ancient names, such as *H. influenzae* Eagan, Rabinowitz (shortened to Rab), or Durst, which are patient names. Flexner also infected monkeys with strains 596, 654, 548. The numbers likely were the lab designations of bacteria other physicians had sent to him, without revealing the patients' names.

Hoping to improve the terrible outcomes, physicians had begun to treat patients with meningitis by subjecting them to repeated spinal taps. The rationale was that by removing the infected cerebrospinal fluid from the patient, the physicians were presumably also removing at least some of the infecting bacteria. The procedure wasn't very effective, if at all.[18] Thus, doctors continued to have no way to treat meningitis. Flexner's intellectual curiosity, as well as "the high mortality of epidemic meningitis and the deplorable deformities caused by it" motivated him to try to "discover therapeutic measures which may mitigate the consequences of the disease."[19(p. 168)]

While studying meningitis in guinea pigs, Flexner hypothesized that the meningococci were so deadly because, during an infection, the bacteria broke apart, liberating their endotoxins,[16] the noxious substances in bacterial membranes originally described two decades earlier by Richard Pfeiffer in cholera-causing bacteria.[20,21] As a possible antidote to the cholera bacteria, Pfeiffer had produced immune serum in guinea pigs by injecting them with *Vibrio cholera*. Even though Pfeiffer's serum didn't kill the cholera bacteria, Flexner figured that immune sera against meningococci might kill the meningococcal bacteria and thus could possibly treat meningitis.[19] This notion was reinforced by Emile Roux's newly described success of antidiphtheria immune serum in treating patients with diphtheria.[22]

The use of immune serum against diphtheria likely began in Germany, and its value became widely known in the scientific community after Roux presented his research in 1894 at the International Medical Congress in Budapest.[23] That same year, two physicians in Cincinnati, Ohio, obtained a small amount of Roux's serum from a colleague who had brought it back from Europe and administered it to a 2-year-old girl with diphtheria. She survived, but two of her siblings, who were not treated, died.[24]

Excitement about the efficacy of diphtheria immune serum in treating diphtheria ran so high that physicians began to treat meningitis with the antidiphtheria serum, in spite of the absence of biologic plausibility that it would work.[25] Even in Flexner's time, scientists recognized that immune serum against the bacteria that caused diphtheria would be of little use against the bacteria that caused meningitis because the therapeutic activity of the serum was specific for each kind of bacteria. But, the doctors were desperate. They would use anything, even a medicine that made no scientific sense, to try to treat children with meningitis.

To confirm his hypothesis that immune serum would treat meningitis, Flexner prepared meningitis immune serum by injecting bacteria from patients in the New York City outbreak into rabbits and goats, obtained blood specimens from the animals, and then separated the colorless serum, which contained antibodies against the meningococci, from the blood's red cells. When he injected the immune serum into animals that were ill from experimentally induced meningitis, the rabbit serum and goat serum successfully treated meningitis in guinea pigs and monkeys, respectively. In fact, Flexner was astonished with the success of the immune serum in treating animals with meningitis; his results greatly exceeded his cautious expectations.[16]

Like most scientists, Flexner was competitive and wanted full credit for discovering the value of his immune sera; in other words, he didn't want to be scooped.[8] When he learned that two groups of scientists in Germany had treated epidemic meningitis patients with immune serum and thus had beaten him in the race to find a treatment, he quickly prepared a preliminary report that described his experiments with meningococcal immune serum in animals.[16] Flexner managed to have the preliminary paper published the same year (1906) that the Germans, Wilhelm Kolle and August von Wassermann[26] and George Jochmann,[27] published their results using meningococcal immune serum to treat humans with meningitis. Thus, Flexner preserved a ray of the limelight for himself. The next year he published a more complete paper of his animal experiments in which he specifically noted his research had begun in 1905, the year the Germans had begun their human experiments. He rather curtly cited the work of the Germans, stating, "The number of [their] cases was too few to permit any conclusion of the value of the injections; but they showed that the injection of horse's serum into the inflamed [spinal] canal [of humans] is not attended with special danger."[19] In the end, Flexner wouldn't acknowledge the therapeutic value of the serum described by the Germans, but he was willing to concede it appeared to be safe.

By the time Flexner had completed his animal experiments with immune sera, the meningitis epidemic in New York had spontaneously subsided, and he no longer had access to a large number of patients to treat with his serum. He began, however, immunizing a horse with meningococci to have large volumes of immune serum for future use.

The description of exactly how he immunized the horse is vague, but he ended up injecting, alternately, live bacteria and lysed bacteria subcutaneously (under their skin).[28] The procedure took months. Ultimately, he immunized three horses and was able to drain 6 liters of serum from each of them every 2 weeks.[29]

Then, yet another epidemic of meningitis struck, this time in January 1907, in Castalia, Ohio, a small town south of Lake Erie's Sandusky Bay. In 4 months, 18 cases of meningitis occurred. As Dr. Louis Ladd described it, "Cerebrospinal meningitis had created such havoc that half the population of the village of six hundred inhabitants fled in terror."[30(p. 1315)] The local physician appealed to the State Board of Health, which put him in touch with Dr. George Crile of Cleveland, who had heard reports of Flexner's serum.[31] Crile arranged for Ladd, an internist from Cleveland, to fetch the serum, along with instructions for its use, from Flexner at the Rockefeller Institute in New York and deliver it to patients in Castalia. Flexner provided his serum free of charge, likely motivated by the altruistic ethics of the time: The care of sick patients trumped everything else. By the time the serum arrived, 3 of the 18 patients were still ill with the infection and were treated. All three fully recovered, for a survival rate of 100%. Of the 15 untreated patients, 12 died, for a survival rate of 20%.[30]

Shortly after the immune serum was used in Castalia, it was given to 11 patients with meningitis in Akron, Ohio, and only 3 died (including 1 patient who was pulseless by the time the treatment was begun), for a survival rate of 75%. Of 9 Akron patients not treated, 8 died, so the survival rate was 11%.[32] The results were certainly promising.

Flexner was cautious, though, about claiming the success of the serum to treat meningitis. Following its use in Akron and Castalia, he wrote,

In order to avoid unnecessary repetition in preparing this discussion [in the scientific paper], some of the above propositions have been stated in a manner that might readily convey the impression that we regard it evident and established that the antiserum has proven its usefulness as a therapeutic agent in epidemic meningitis. The facts of our belief, at the present time, are quite otherwise. No one could be less convinced of the final fact of its value than we are.[28(p. 202)]

Word that the serum was successful, however, spread rapidly,[13] and Flexner was hesitant to share the serum with physicians who might not use it appropriately. He told the Suffolk District Medical Society in Boston,

> You see therefore that it will be impossible for us to send the serum to all of those who ask for it. It seems best to guard its use rather carefully while we are in the experimental stage. ... Therefore I am especially anxious that the serum should be in the hands of a few observers of first-rate critical judgment.[29(p. 387)]

Despite Flexner's caution, he made his serum available to a number of physicians. In Cleveland, Ladd ultimately treated 13 patients; 5 died, for a survival rate of 64%.[30] In Washington, D.C., the survival rate was 70%, and in Philadelphia, it was 80%.[13]

In Porterville, California, a town of 2,000 inhabitants at the foot of the Sierra Nevada Mountains in the San Joaquin Valley, the survival rate of treated patients was 84%, compared to 8% among untreated patients.[33] In Boston and surrounding towns, the survival rate of patients treated by Charles Dunn was 75%. In describing his surviving patients, Dunn summarized the three major effects of the treatment: (1) The fever rapidly resolved (Figure 6.4); (2) the general condition of the

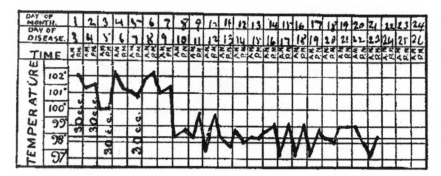

FIGURE 6.4 Resolution of fever two days after the last treatment with immune serum in a patient with epidemic meningitis. The four doses of meningococcal antiserum are indicated beneath the fever curve for days of the month 1, 2, 3, and 5.

From Dunn CH. The Serum Treatment of Epidemic Cerebrospinal Meningitis. *Journal of the American Medical Association.* 1908;51:15–21.

patients rapidly improved; and (3) all meningeal symptoms subsided, with few sequelae.[18]

Although different protocols were used to administer the antiserum, it was always given directly into the patients' lumbar (lower back) spinal column (Figure 6.5). Usually, up to 30 mL of spinal fluid were first removed, and then the serum was injected. Most patients received between 30 and 45 mL with each injection, and many received daily injections for 4 days, some even longer.[18]

By 1913, Flexner's serum had been used around the world, and the survival rates of epidemic meningitis had improved from 10% to 30% among the untreated to 70% among those treated with the immune serum (Figure 6.6). The earlier in the course of the infection it was given, the better the outcome was.[14]

During his study of the bacteria isolated from the patients with epidemic meningitis, Flexner learned that meningococcal strains were not all alike. They differed in their ability to cause illness in animals, in their ability to be digested by white blood cells, and in their ability to disintegrate when mixed with immune serum. Further, a few patients didn't respond to the serum treatment at all. Meningococcal strains recovered from those poor responders seemed "fast" to the serum, in that they were resistant to being broken apart and were not killed when mixed with immune serum.[14] Thus, something, a mysterious, unknown factor, was different in some of the strains.

In preparing his immune serum, Flexner had used several (an undescribed number) bacterial strains to immunize the horses, thus improving the probability that the resultant serum would be effective against strains that exhibited the mysterious differences he had observed. A likely candidate for the "unknown factor" was the capsule of meningococci, which was discovered in 1909 by the French physician Charles Dopter during his experiments on the serologic differences in strains.[34] The meningococcal capsule was systematically characterized between 1915 and 1918.[35] Now we know that meningococci have 13 immunologically distinct capsules (or, like *H. influenzae*, they may also have no capsule), and serogroups A, B, C, X, Y, and W bacteria are capable of infecting humans. Most infections in North America are

APPARATUS FOR INJECTING ANTI-MENINGITIS SERUM.

This special gravity container has been devised by Mr. E. R. Alexander, formerly of the Research Laboratory of New York, and the Author, with the purpose of supplying the serum in a condition ready for use in a sealed aseptic container with sterile apparatus easy to assemble with little manipulation. It is especially adapted for the superior and safer gravity method for administering the antimeningitis serum.

DIRECTIONS FOR USE.

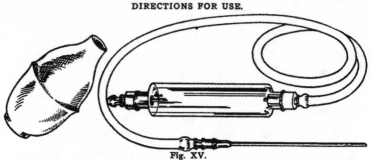

Fig. XV.

1. After making lumbar puncture remove the trocar "B" from needle "A" and allow the cerebrospinal fluid to escape.

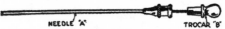

NEEDLE "A"   TROCAR "B"

Fig. XVI.

2. Plunge stylet "C" attached to rubber tubing through the hole in rubber stopper of container at end "D" until the bead in the stopper is dislodged.

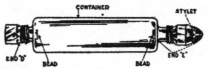

CONTAINER   STYLET

END "D"   BEAD   BEAD   END "E"

Fig. XVII.

3. Remove capping skin from end "E" and similarly plunge stylet already attached until bead is dislodged and the flow will be started.
4. When serum appears at the end "F" of rubber tube attach the latter to the needle.
5. Control the rate of flow by raising or lowering the serum container.

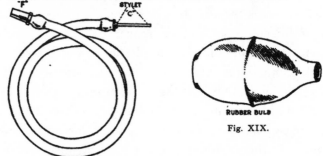

"F"   STYLET "C"

RUBBER BULB

Fig. XIX.

Fig. XVIII.

6. If the serum does not flow well, the bulb may be attached to the upper stylet at end "E" and the necessary pressure slowly exerted. This procedure is not advised, however, since under normal conditions the flow runs well by gravity alone.

N. B. See that the beads, which are in the holes in rubber stopper at each end of the container are dislodged. If they adhere to ends of stylets a gentle shaking will quickly dislodge them.

FIGURE 6.5 Apparatus for injecting antimeningitis serum into the spinal canal of patients.

From Sophian A. *Epidemic Cerebrospinal Meningitis.* St. Louis, MO: Mosby; 1913:210.

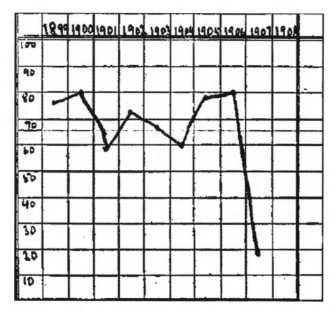

FIGURE 6.6 Mortality rates of patients with meningococcal meningitis at Children's Hospital in Boston from 1899 to 1907. Treatment with meningococcal antiserum began in 1907.

From Dunn CH. The Serum Treatment of Epidemic Cerebrospinal Meningitis. *Journal of the American Medical Association.* 1908;51:15–21.

caused by serogroups B and C, while serogroup A is most common in the "meningitis belt" of sub-Saharan Africa.

Not everyone, however, was thrilled about Flexner's immune serum. Members of the New York Anti-Vivisection Society demanded cessation of the animal experiments at the Rockefeller Institute. The reaction against the legislation proposed to the New York legislature by the anti-vivisectionists, however, was swift and loud. One motherwrote,

> There is not one woman in New York who would not hail with enthusiasm the barest chance of saving her own child's life, or of lessening its suffering, by the sacrifice of any animal, big or little; and yet, when the question arises of applying the much discussed doctrine of vivisection to the help of suffering humanity at large, there goes up a wail of tender-hearted protest against the heartless and

needless pain inflicted on the poor, dumb beasts, and this in face of the fact that statistics prove the immense benefit derived by human sufferers as the direct result of the skilled and merciful experiments which our highest medical men have been carrying on.[36(p. 333)]

Even Mrs. Cadwallader Jones, the president of the Women's Auxiliary of the American Society for the Prevention of Cruelty to Animals, recognizing the practical utility of animal immune serum in treating meningitis in children, opposed the legislative measure, stating "the regulations at present in force in regard to vivisection are ample to provide against abuses in its practice."[36(p. 333)]

The physicians who injected immune serum into patients to treat meningitis soon learned it was not without peril. In that regard, meningitis antiserum was similar to the diphtheria antitoxin previously used, without benefit, to treat meningitis, as both resulted in adverse reactions that included fevers, rashes, joint pains, or swelling. The serum was, after all, obtained from horses, and the immune systems of living animals, including humans, protect themselves from invaders by developing antibodies against foreign substances. When the meningitis patients were injected with the horse serum that contained a number of horse proteins, many of them developed antibodies against that foreign serum and experienced subsequent symptoms, called serum sickness.

Rufus Cole reviewed the negative effects related to injections of horse immune serum and identified three types:

1. Anaphylaxis, a severe immune reaction that occurred immediately following the second dose of serum (the first dose had "sensitized" the patients so they developed antibodies against the horse serum, and after the second dose of horse serum, the antibodies from the sensitization dose bound to the horse proteins in the second dose and caused the reactions). Anaphylaxis resulted in redness of the face, restlessness, increased heart rate, difficulty in breathing, urticaria (hives), and, rarely, cardiovascular collapse.
2. A reaction, which could occur after the first dose of antiserum, with clinical manifestations similar to anaphylaxis but the result of

contaminants in the horse serum rather than to antibodies against the horse proteins; these effects varied from lot to lot of the serum.

3. Serum sickness, which occurred 4 to 14 days after the treatment. This reaction, which resulted in fever, skin rashes, gland swelling, skin edema, and arthritis, was caused by immune complexes composed of antibodies plus the bacteria (or bacterial fragments) to which the antibodies bound.[37] The immune complexes circulated through the blood to many organs and became trapped in their tiny capillaries, causing the resultant symptoms.

Flexner had seen such reactions to the horse serum in his animal experiments[16] and decided that delivery of the serum to humans directly into their spinal columns would offer three advantages, as it would (1) bypass the blood; (2) deliver the antibodies to the site of the infection; and (3) reduce the adverse symptoms. He seemed to be correct, as the patients treated with his immune horse serum experienced few reactions.

The year Flexner accepted his research position at the Rockefeller University, 1903, he married Helen Whithall Thomas. She was the daughter of an Evangelist mother and a Quaker father whose family of British origin had been in America for many generations. Helen's father was a trustee of Johns Hopkins University, and her sister Carey became the president of Bryn Mawr College, where Helen became a professor of English.[6] It was Helen who opened Simon's mind to the arts, and ancient Chinese paintings became his favorite genre. Helen and Simon had two sons, William Welch Flexner, a mathematics professor, and James Thomas Flexner, a historian.[38]

With the opening of the Rockefeller Institute, Simon became its first director. He was by nature enthusiastic, impulsive, shy, and high strung, and yet, as a leader, he exhibited "a serenity that verged on fortitude." As written by his admirer Peyton Rous,

One of his best strengths was a logic far beyond that of most men, final as a knife; and, acting as this logic directed, he became able in time to dismiss worries because they should be dismissed, and to arrive at decisions without any mental gesticulations or strayings. ... To watch him ... was to watch a perfectly tooled mind in action.[6(p. 426)]

Flexner continued to direct the Rockefeller Institute until, seeking quiet and simplicity, he retired at age 72. He died of a heart attack in New York on May 2, 1946, at age 83.

While Flexner clearly demonstrated the benefit of meningococcal immune sera in treating epidemic meningitis, information on the ability of immune sera to treat meningitis caused by other bacteria such as pneumococci and *H. influenzae* was much slower to come. Compared to epidemic meningitis caused by meningococci, the mortality rates for meningitis patients infected with the other bacteria were particularly awful.

Among 631 patients with well-documented pneumococcal meningitis, only 1 patient survived.[39] After immune serum was shown to improve the outcomes of patients with pneumococcal pneumonia,[37] numerous case reports using immune sera to treat *Streptococcus pneumoniae* meningitis appeared in the medical literature. In the first such report, 14 patients were treated, and, although transient improvement may have occurred, none of the patients survived.[40] Several case reports, however, suggested benefit using pneumococcal immune serum, but many scientists doubted their validity because the authors failed to include credible bacteriologic data to confirm the causes of the infections.[41,42] One difficulty using serum to treat pneumococcal meningitis was the many serotypes of *S. pneumoniae*; currently, almost a hundred have been identified.[43] Thus, to have any hope of therapeutic efficacy, the serum used to treat a patient with pneumococcal meningitis would have to be specific for the serotype of the strain causing that infection, and the complex logistics of this therapeutic approach were insurmountable.

After the success of meningococcal immune sera to treat meningococcal meningitis, many physicians sought a similar treatment for *H. influenzae* meningitis because it was more deadly than meningococcal meningitis, with mortality rates in young children well above 90%.[44,45] Flexner himself speculated that the many deaths from influenzal meningitis could possibly be averted by treating the patients with influenzal antisera, that is, immune sera made against *H. influenzae* bacteria.[46] *Haemophilus influenzae* meningitis, however, did not occur in epidemics, so treatment trials couldn't focus on outbreaks or clusters of cases as had been done with meningococcal immune sera, but, rather, had to be conducted one isolated case at a time.

Dr. Martha Wollstein, who had tried to understand the confusing immune reactions of *H. influenzae* and was strongly influenced by Flexner's work with serum therapy for meningococcal meningitis, was the first to experiment with anti-influenzal serum to treat children with *H. influenzae* meningitis. To prepare the serum, she immunized a goat by injecting it with live *H. influenzae* "over intervals" for 18 months. Initially, she injected bacteria isolated from the respiratory tract of an unnamed child, but after 2 months, the immunized goat had not developed any evidence of an immunologic response. Subsequently she continued to immunize the goat with "virulent" *H. influenzae*. The goat immediately developed agglutinating and opsonic antibodies, indicating a vigorous immune response. As proof of principle that influenzal serum would treat influenzal meningitis, she infected three monkeys by injecting *H. influenzae* she had scraped from "two slant cultures" (a very large number of bacteria) into their cerebrospinal fluids by lumbar puncture, and 1 to 24 hours later she treated the infected monkeys with the goat serum, again by lumbar puncture. It worked. All of the animals were cured "after very severe [albeit brief] disease."[47]

Next Wollstein used the goat serum to treat three children with influenzal meningitis. It failed. All three children died, but she was encouraged that before death, their clinical conditions had improved somewhat, presumably in response to the serum.[48]

Others also tried Wollstein's goat anti-influenzal serum. Dr. Josephine Neal treated five patients with influenzal serum, and one survived. Neal couldn't credit the serum with the recovery, though, as that patient had received multiple spinal taps (which had occasionally been thought to promote recovery). In addition, the patient had been treated with both several doses of "stock vaccine," which presumably was the bacterial concoction used to vaccinate the horses from which the immune serum was harvested, and "autogenous vaccine," which presumably was made from the patient's own bacteria.[49] Dr. Charles Hunter Dunn, however, treated 11 cases with influenzal immune serum, and none survived. Dunn acknowledged that all his patients received the serum late in the courses of their infections—probably too late for it to possibly be effective.[50]

Lack of success of the influenzal immune serum treatment discouraged its further use until 1932, when Drs. Leroy Fothergill (of the famous microbiology graph fame) and Hugh Ward in Boston recognized that influenzal meningitis was more common than previously realized, possibly because diseases of adults dominated medical thinking at the time. In addition, influenzal meningitis was associated with high mortality. Thus, Fothergill and Ward began to explore influenzal immune serum as treatment. Interestingly, although they had learned of Wollstein's failures in treating influenzal meningitis in monkeys with serum, they stated they could "find no record of the use of this serum in human infections. Our attempts [to find such cases] go back several years."[51(p. 874)] They apparently hadn't searched the medical literature back far enough, though, for the previous reports that used Wollstein's goat serum in children (some likely didn't have *H. influenzae* type b meningitis) were published more than a decade prior to their own work.[49,50,52,53]

In an attempt to improve the outcome of patients treated with *H. influenzae* immune serum, Fothergill and Ward finally altered their serum treatment protocol based on reports that cerebrospinal fluid lacked complement, the protein that enhances the effect of antibodies. When they added complement to the horse immune serum in their laboratory experiments, the serum killed *H. influenzae* more effectively. They also noted the Neisser-Wechsberg phenomenon (also called the antibody prozone phenomenon), in which highly concentrated immune serum did not kill bacteria while diluted serum did. They concluded that the proportion of antibodies relative to complement was important for optimal bacterial killing.[51,54]

Ward and Wright then treated eight patients with immune serum mixed with complement, but the results, unfortunately, weren't good—only one of the patients survived. They considered altering the protocol yet again, but humbly stated, "It must be admitted that so far we have not had the courage to advise a change in the proportion of antiserum to complement. ... Most of the cases responded favourably at first [although seven of the eight ultimately died] and one has to be very sure of a theory to change a treatment under these conditions."[55(p. 230)]

Others had also noted temporary clinical improvement and temporary sterilization of the cerebrospinal fluid in patients treated with the influenzal immune antisera, only to be followed by the patients' deaths.[45,49,56] On autopsy of patients treated with influenzal immune sera, Ward and Wright found abscesses in the infected brains and concluded that the antibodies present in the immune serum were unable to penetrate the walls of the abscess to treat the bacteria inside, resulting in its failure to cure the infection.[51]

In spite of their initial dismal results, Fothergill and his colleagues nevertheless persisted in treating influenzal meningitis patients with their horse influenzal immune serum as no alternative treatments were shown to be effective. Their protocol consisted of draining all the spinal fluid from the patient by lumbar puncture, running two parts serum plus one part complement (the antibody-enhancer protein from blood), for a total of 23 mL, into the spinal canal by gravity and then elevating the foot of the bed for an hour, presumably to allow the serum in cerebrospinal fluid to run downhill and thus to accumulate more quickly in the brain. The treatments were administered twice a day "for as long as is indicated." In considering the optimal duration of the serum therapy, Fothergill wrote,

> In those patients that are recovering, it is difficult to decide when to stop treatment. This must be decided for each individual case from a careful consideration of all the evidence that yields information regarding the course of the disease. [This] and [the patient's] response to therapy is best obtained by a daily examination of the cerebrospinal fluid. A fall in the total cell count, a return of sugar to the normal amount and an increase in the percentage of mononuclear cells is evidence of improvement.[57(p. 589)]

Compared to no treatment, Fothergill's serum therapy in patients with influenzal meningitis resulted in only slight improvement in survival: 31 of 201 patients lived, for a survival rate of 15.4%. He thought the poor outcome was related to the brain abscesses he also had observed in the patients who had died and to the much higher numbers of bacteria in the influenzal patients' cerebrospinal fluid compared to that of patients with meningococcal meningitis.

Another possible explanation might be related to the influenzal strains Fothergill used to produce the antiserum. Even if the strains used to immunize the horse originally possessed a capsule (which wasn't discovered by Margaret Pittman until after Fothergill's experiments), the capsules may have been lost during the repeated culturing of the strains on agar, which was necessary to keep the bacteria alive.[55] In that case, the immune serum wouldn't have contained antibodies against the capsule, now known to be the most important component of protective *H. influenzae* antiserum.

The experiments conducted by Fothergill and Ward were expensive. They immunized several horses, which had to be housed and fed. They had to buy agar and other ingredients for the media to grow their bacteria. They needed glassware, which had to be manually washed and sterilized after each use. They needed microscopes, refrigerators, freezers, incubators, autoclaves, and technicians to assist with the experiments. In Fothergill and Ward's paper, the authors acknowledged the cost of their work and stated, "At this stage it became possible, largely owing to the establishment of the Philip Ellis Stevens, Jr. Memorial Fund, for the study of this disease [influenzal meningitis], to investigate the problem more thoroughly."[51(p. 875)]

Who, one wonders, was Philip Ellis Stevens, Jr.? An Internet search reveals the gravestone in Nashua, New Hampshire, of such a person who was born April 5, 1927, and died November 28, 1929, at age two and a half years.[58] The child's father, Philip Ellis Stevens, Sr., of Nashua, New Hampshire, was a successful businessman[59] and likely a man of means. Little Philip from neighboring New Hampshire could have been a patient at Boston's Infant's and Children's Hospital, where Fothergill and Ward worked. None of the patients described in their research papers, however, match with Philip's initials, age, or gender. The Stevens memorial gift is cited as funding the research of the Ward, Fothergill, and Wright group from 1932 to 1937. We can speculate that little Philip's parents appreciated the care their son received and thus established the memorial gift to further research on the disease that so tragically took their child from them, and that the Fothergill group, likely always short on funds, greatly appreciated their generosity.

On Pittman's discovery of the six capsules of *H. influenzae*[60] and recognition that most cases of meningitis were due to strains carrying the type b capsule, immune serum could be developed that was specific for type b strains. Pittman did just that. She immunized a horse—the procedure took over 2 years to complete—with 27 different type b strains, carefully documenting that each strain was the "S," or Smooth, slimy variety that possessed a capsule. When she infected mice and rabbits with *H. influenzae* and then treated them with her horse immune serum, their outcomes were improved over those of untreated animals. Reassured by these results, she studied the effect of her serum on children with *H. influenzae* meningitis.

Pittman herself was a microbiologist rather than a physician, and the Rockefeller Hospital where she worked cared only for adults, so she enlisted a cadre of pediatricians from the New York area to treat their patients with her serum. Ultimately, 13 children, ranging in age from 2 months to 7 years, with documented type b *H. influenzae* meningitis received Pittman's serum, along with fresh serum to provide added complement, but under varying clinical circumstances and using varying infusion protocols. Only one survived.

Thus, hope that patients with influenzal meningitis would benefit from treatment with influenzal immune serum, even type b–specific serum, was cruelly dashed. While immune serum had dramatically improved the outcome of patients with epidemic meningitis caused by meningococci, it just didn't work against *H. influenzae* infection. Dorothy Wilkes-Weiss and Robert Huntington finally rang the death knell: "In conclusion, it may be stated that the results of serum treatment of influenzal meningitis have been discouraging, and that there is no obvious justification for optimism as to the possibilities of future work. The use of such serum is purely experimental, and its commercial exploitation seems quite unjustified."[45](p. 465)

References

1. Flexner S, Barker LF. The Recent Outbreak of Epidemic Cerebro-Spinal Meningitis at Lonaconing and Other Places in the Valley of George's Creek, Maryland. *Bulletin of the Johns Hopkins Hospital.* 1893;4(32):68–71.
2. Flexner S, Barker LF. A Contribution to Our Knowledge of Epidemic Cerebro-Spinal Meningitis. *The American Journal of the Medical Sciences.* 1894;107(Feb–Mar):155–172, 259–276.
3. Weichselbaum A. Ueber die Aetiologie der Akuten Meningitis Cerebrospinalis. *Fortschritte der Medizin.* 1887;5:573–583.

4. Ligon BL. Albert Ludwig Sigesmund Neisser: Discoverer of the Cause of Gonorrhea. *Seminars in Pediatric Infectious Diseases.* 2005;16(4):336–341.

5. Neisser A. Uber eine der Gonorrhoe eigentumliche Mikrokokkusform. Vorlaufige mitteilung. *Zentralblatt fur die Medizinischen Wissenschraften* 1879;17(28):497–500.

6. Rous P. Simon Flexner. 1863–1946. *Obituary Notices of Fellows of the Royal Society.* 1949;6(18):408–445.

7. Flexner JT. *An American Saga: The Story of Helen Thomas and Simon Flexner.* New York: Fordham University Press; 1993.

8. Artenstein AW. *In the Blink of an Eye: The Deadly Story of Epidemic Meningitis.* Berlin: Springer Science+Business; 2012.

9. Prudden TM. *The Story of the Bacteria and Their Relations to Health and Disease.* New York: Putnam's Sons; 1889.

10. Flexner A. *Medical Education in the United States and Canada: A Report to the Carnegie Foundation for the Advancement of Teaching.* New York: Carnegie Foundation; 1910.

11. Billings JSJ. Cerebrospinal Meningitis in New York City During 1904 and 1905. *Journal of the American Medical Association.* 1906;46(22):1670–1676.

12. Burton Hendrick, Historian, 78, Dies. *New York Times,* March 25, 1949.

13. Hendrick BJ. Conquering Spinal Meningitis: What the Rockefeller Institute Has Done for Children. *McClure's Magazine.* 1909;32:594–603.

14. Flexner S. The Results of the Serum Treatment in Thirteen Hundred Cases of Epidemic Meningitis. *The Journal of Experimental Medicine.* 1913;17(5):553–576.

15. Flexner S. Contributions to the Biology of *Diplococcus intracellularis. The Journal of Experimental Medicine.* 1907;9(2):105–141.

16. Flexner S. Experimental Cerebrospinal Meningitis and Its Serum Treatment. *Journal of the American Medical Association.* 1906;47(8):560–566.

17. Flexner S. Experimental Cerebro-Spinal Meningitis in Monkeys. *The Journal of Experimental Medicine.* 1907;9(2):142–141.

18. Dunn CH. The Serum Treatment of Epidemic Cerebrospinal Meningitis. *Journal of the American Medical Association.* 1908;51(1):15–21.

19. Flexner S. Concerning a Serum-Therapy for Experimental Infection with *Diplococcus intracellularis. The Journal of Experimental Medicine.* 1907;9(2):168–185.

20. Pfeiffer R. Weitere Mitteilungen über die Spezifischen Antikörper der Cholera. *Zeitschrift für Hygiene.* 1894;18:1–16.

21. Rietschel ET, Cavaillon JM. Richard Pfeiffer and Alexandre Besredka: Creators of the Concept of Endotoxin and Anti-endotoxin. *Microbes and Infection.* 2003;5(15):1407–1414.

22. Roux E, Martin L, Chaillou A. Trois Cents cas de Diphterie Traites par le Serum Antidiphterique. *Annales de l'Institut Pasteur.* 1894;8:640–661.

23. Nuttall GHF, Loeffler FAJ, Graham-Smith GS. *The Bacteriology of Diphtheria Including Sections on the History, Epidemiology and Pathology*

of the Disease, the Mortality Caused by It, the Toxins and Antitoxins and the Serum Disease. Cambridge, England: Cambridge University Press; 1908.

24. Youngdahl K. Early Use of Diphtheria Antitoxin in the United States. *The History of Vaccines.* 2010. http://www.historyofvaccines.org/content/blog/early-uses-diphtheria-antitoxin-united-states. Accessed November 14, 2016.

25. Dunn CH. The Serum Treatment of Epidemic Cerebrospinal Meningitis. *Boston Medical and Surgical Journal.* 1908;158(12):370–179.

26. Kolle W, Wassermann A. Versuche zur Gewinnung und Wertbestimmung eines Meningococcenserums. *Deutsche medizinische Wochenschrift.* 1906;32(16):609–612.

27. Jochmann G. Versuche zur Serodiagnostik und Serotherapie der Epidemischen Genickstarre. *Deutsche medizinische Wochenschrift.* 1906;33:788–793.

28. Flexner S, Jobling JW. Serum Treatment of Epidemic Cerebro-Spinal Meningitis. *The Journal of Experimental Medicine.* 1908;10(1):141–203.

29. Cabot RC. The Suffolk District Medical Society Meeting. *Boston Medical and Surgical Journal.* 1908;158(12):384–387.

30. Ladd LW. Serum Treatment of Epidemic Cerebro-Spinal Meningitis. *Journal of the American Medical Association.* 1908;51(16):1315–1318.

31. Storey W. Cerebro-Spinal Fever in Castalia and Vicinity. *Ohio State Medical Journal.* 1906–1907;2:674–676.

32. Chase WS, Hunt ML. Serotherapy of Epidemic Cerebrospinal Meningitis. *Archives of Internal Medicine.* 1908;1:294–313.

33. Miller A, Barber SA. An Epidemic of Cerebrospinal Meningitis and the Successful Use of Flexner's Antiserum. *Journal of the American Medical Association.* 1908;50(24):1975–1977.

34. Dopter C. Etude de Quelques Germes Isoles du Rhinopharynx Voisins du Meningococcque (para Meningocoques). *Comptes Rendus des Seances de la Societe de Biologie. (Paris).* 1909;67:74–76.

35. Branham SE. Milestones in the History of the Meningococcus. *Canadian Journal of Microbiology.* 1956;2(3):175–188.

36. The Rockefeller Institute and Antivivisection. *Boston Medical and Surgical Journal.* 1908;158(10):333.

37. Cole R. Report of Studies Concerning Acute Lobar Pneumonia. *Journal of the American Medical Association.* 1917;69(7):505–508.

38. Institute for Advanced Study: Past member, William Welch Flexner. https://www.ias.edu/scholars/william-welch-flexner. Accessed July 22, 2019.

39. Waring GW, Weinstein L. The Treatment of Pneumococcal Meningitis. *The American Journal of the Medicine.* 1948;5(3):402–418.

40. Litchfield L. Abstract of Discussion. *Journal of the American Medical Association.* 1917;69(7):508–509.

41. Harkavy J. Pneumococcus Meningitis: Recovery with Serum Therapy. *Journal of the American Medical Association.* 1928;90(8):597–599.

42. Vogelius H. Pneumococcal Meningitis Treated with Specific Serum and Chemotherapeutic Drugs of the Sulphanilamide Group—4 Cases of Recovery. *Acta Medica Scandinavica.* 1941;106(5–6):449–467.

43. Geno KA, Gilbert GL, Song JY, et al. Pneumococcal Capsules and Their Types: Past, Present, and Future. *Clinical Microbiology Reviews.* 2015;28(3):871–899.

44. Rivers TM. Influenzal Meningitis. *American Journal of Diseases of Children.* 1922;24(2):102–124.

45. Wilkes-Weiss D, Huntington RW Jr. The Treatment of Influenzal Meningitis with Immune Serum. *The Journal of Pediatrics.* 1936;9(4):462–466.

46. Flexner S. Influenzal Meningitis and Its Serum Treatment. *Journal of the American Medical Association.* 1911;57(1):16–16.

47. Wollstein M. Serum Treatment of Influenzal Meningitis. *Journal of Experimental Medicine.* 1911;14(1):73–82.

48. Wollstein M. Influenzal Meningitis: Experimental and Clinical. *Transactions of the Fifteenth International Congress of Hygiene and Demography, 1912.* 1913;2(Pt. 1):57–62.

49. Neal JB. Influenzal Meningitis. *Archives of Pediatrics.* 1921 38(1):1–10.

50. Dunn CH, Rotch TM. *Pediatrics, the Hygienic and Medical Treatment of Children.* Troy, NY: Southworth; 1922.

51. Ward HK, Fothergill LD. Influenzal Meningitis Treated with Specific Antiserum and Complement. *American Journal of Diseases of Childhood.* 1932;43(4):873–881.

52. Torrey RG. Influenzal Meningitis, with Report of a Case. *The American Journal of the Medical Sciences.* 1916;152:403–410.

53. Packard FR. Report of a Case of Acute Mastoiditis with Influenzal Meningitis. Treatment by Operation on the Mastoid and Antiinfluenzal Serum, Followed by Brain Abscess—Operation. *The Annals of Otology, Rhinology & Laryngology.* 1916;25:706–709.

54. Kolmer JA. The Mechanism of Immunologic Changes in the Cerebrospinal Fluid. *Archives of Neurology & Psychiatry.* 1925;14(2):233–239.

55. Ward HK, Wright J. Studies on Influenzal Meningitis: I. The Problems of Specific Therapy. *The Journal of Experimental Medicine.* 1932;55(2):223–234.

56. Pittman M. The Action of Type-Specific *Hemophilus influenzae* Antiserum. *The Journal of Experimental Medicine.* 1933;58(6):683–706.

57. Fothergill LRD. *Hemophilus influenzae* (Pfeiffer Bacillus) Meningitis and Its Specific Treatment. *New England Journal of Medicine.* 1937;216(14):587–590.

58. Billion Graves. Philip Ellis Stevens Jr. https://pl.billiongraves.com/grave/Philip-Ellis-Stevens-Jr/1548338#/. Accessed December 1, 2016.

59. We Would Like to Express to All Our Customers and Friends. *Nashua Telegraph.* December 31, 1959. https://www.newspapers.com/newspage/74733871/. Accessed December 1, 2016.

60. Pittman M. Variation and Type Specificity in the Bacterial Species *Hemophilus influenzae*. *The Journal of Experimental Medicine.* 1931;53(4):471–492.

7

Antibiotic Treatment—Much Better than Nothing

DURING THE AGE OF antiquity, meningitis was an enigmatic illness, a disease surrounded by myths and magic, wizardry and folklore. Its symptoms, like those of all illnesses, were considered by Hippocrates to be an imbalance of the four bodily humors: phlegm, blood, yellow bile, and black bile. Seizures, a common manifestation of meningitis, were thought to be a curse, a punishment from the gods.[1] As far as fever was concerned, William Cullen, the Scottish physician and author of *First Lines of the Practice of Physic*, attributed its proximal cause to debility in the state of the animal system (although Cullen's definition of animal system is vague, he likely meant physiologic equilibrium), resulting in diminished energy of the brain.[2] Cullen credited the remote cause of fever to miasmata arising from marshes or moist ground that is acted on by heat. Even after meningitis had been accurately described as a bacterial infection, death from meningitis was said to be caused by a black cat (or the shadow of a black cat) running between the patient's parents.[3]

While the perplexing symptoms befuddled and frightened both old-time physicians and the families of its victims, the treatment of meningitis remained obscure for a very long time. The patients writhed, quaked, slept, didn't respond to questions or pain, and finally died, and no one knew, with certainty, how to cure it. As described by Juan Sorapán de Rieros and José Sbarbi in 1876, the treatment for meningitis, along with other maladies, in Spain involved preparing a poultice

Continual Raving: A History of Meningitis and the People Who Conquered It. Janet R Gilsdorf, Oxford University Press (2020). © Oxford University Press.
DOI: 10.1093/oso/9780190677312.001.0001

by opening a freshly killed small animal, such as a toad, dove, pigeon, frog, sheep, or chicken, and then rubbing the bloody inside of the creature on the patient's body.[4,5] In the days of Dr. John Cooke, early in the nineteenth century, treatments for hydrocephalus (a complication of meningitis) included a) purging; b) blood-letting; c) blisters [applications of, derived from the blister beetle (or Spanish fly), to the skin, which resulted in a blister to draw out evil humors[6]]; d) setons and issues [skin breaks, often created by a needle, scalpel, or lancet and accompanied by the insertion of a thread or other foreign object to allow evil humors to drain[7]]; e) revellents ["agents [that] by producing a modified action in some organ or texture, derive from the morbid condition of some other organ or texture"[8(p. 333)]], such as emetics, blisters, irritants; f) refrigerants externally applied and certain medicines taken internally, which are supposed to produce a specific effect, particularly mercury; and g) corroborants [agents that are invigorating, such as Peruvian bark, wine, or dogwood[9]] and sedatives, especially [chinchoa or Peruvian] bark and opium.[10]

By the early twentieth century, treatments for meningitis had evolved to include repeated lumbar punctures to drain off the offending bacteria; diphtheria antitoxin, even though the bacteria that caused diphtheria didn't cause meningitis; and infusions of immune sera into the subdural space to deliver immune factors directly to the infection. None worked, other than Flexner's immune serum for meningococcal meningitis. The patients kept dying.

In the evening of May 16, 1935, when Katherine Woglom, a healthy 10-year-old, suddenly became ill, her parents, Dr. and Mrs. William W. Woglom, took her, reportedly their only child, to Willard Parker Hospital in New York City. At the time of her admission, she was semicomatose. The doctors examined her airway with a laryngoscope and saw the telltale signs of epiglottitis (inflammation of the epiglottis, the tissue that flips over the windpipe during swallowing to prevent food from descending into the lungs). The swollen epiglottis obstructed the flow of air into her lungs, so her doctors performed an emergency tracheostomy to facilitate her ability to breathe. Six days later, her breathing had improved, and the tracheostomy tube was removed, but she continued to have a fever and, after 12 more days, developed a stiff neck. Her doctors performed a spinal tap, and the fluid showed elevated protein and increased white blood cells (580/mm^3). These findings were consistent with bacterial meningitis, but no bacteria were recovered. Four days later, *Haemophilus influenzae* grew from her blood culture, indirectly confirming she had *H. influenzae* meningitis.[11]

Katherine was transferred to Babies' Hospital in New York 3 weeks into her illness, and a second spinal tap revealed increased white blood cells (1,100/mm^3, with 60% neutrophils); elevated protein (80 mg/ 100 mL); and decreased glucose (30 mg/100 mL) in the spinal fluid. Again, these findings were consistent with bacterial meningitis, but, again, no bacteria grew from the cerebrospinal fluid specimen. At that time, Katherine was fully conscious and extremely apprehensive. Over the next 10 days, her mental status deteriorated, and she developed papilledema (swelling of the optic nerves at the back of her eyeballs), indicating increased pressure inside her head. Her condition was considered grave.

While Katherine, feverish and unresponsive, languished in her hospital bed, her despondent physician father scoured the medical literature for something, anything, that might help his daughter. On July 8, he ran across news of a novel aniline dye, Prontosil (also known as sulfachrysoidine), that had been used to treat bacterial infections in Germany. He immediately told Katherine's primary physician, Dr. Ashley Weech, about the dye. Weech hurried to the hospital library and found the July copy of the German medical journal *Deutsche medizinische Wochenschrift*, which contained not one, but four articles from Bayer Laboratories and several hospitals in Germany reporting the success of the red dye sulfachrysoidine in treating streptococcal infections.[12–15] How Weech translated the papers isn't known. But, after recognizing their importance, Weech called Dr. Frank Stockman, the medical director of Winthrop Laboratories (an American subsidiary of Bayer Laboratories), who said that the first shipment of Prontosil had arrived just that day from Germany. Stockman sent a small amount of the drug to Weech (Figure 7.1).

Both Woglom and Weech knew the risks. Very few patients had been treated with the dye, and none of them had *H. influenzae* meningitis. Surely the drug would have side effects, and these were unknown to them. The supply of the drug was very limited. They had no idea how

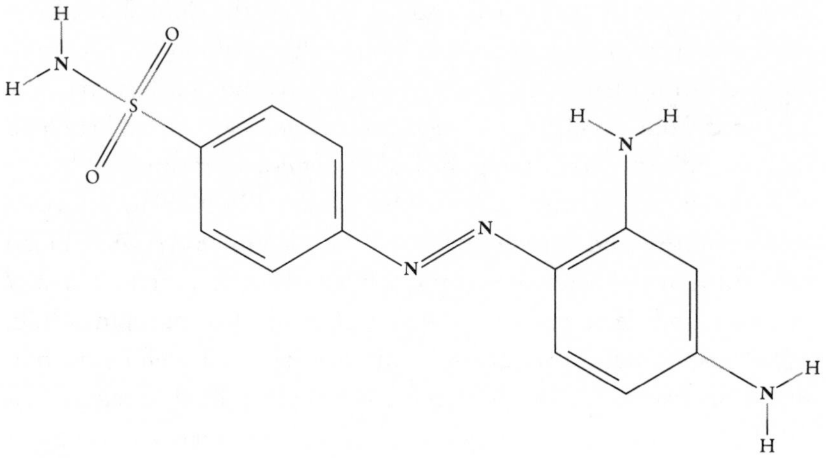

FIGURE 7.1 Chemical structure of Prontosil.
From National Center for Biochemistry Information (PubChem). https://pubchem. ncbi.nlm.nih.gov/compound/prontosil#section=Top.

much of the dye to give to a child with meningitis. And yet, Katherine was deathly ill. On July 10, Weech ordered the drug to be given, and that afternoon, the chief pediatric resident, Dr. Howell Wright, pushed 10 mL of the dye, the color of well-aged burgundy, into Katherine's vein though a hypodermic needle. She received the drug twice a day for 5 days and then three times a day for 8 days more.

By 2 days after the first dose, Katherine's color had improved, and she looked somewhat better. Her neurologic symptoms, though, showed no improvement. Her neck was still stiff, and her optic discs were still swollen. By July 21, she continued to have fever, and the papilledema had increased. She picked at her nose constantly without purpose and episodically stared at the wall, apparently without seeing. Weech con- cluded that these symptoms supported the presence of a brain abscess. His note in her medical record that day read,

> The change [possible improvement in her condition], however, has not been dramatic, not even progressive, and it is difficult to exclude coincidence in the relation between therapy and change. My own feeling is that Prontosil has not done a great deal. I would never- theless wish to try it again—if the present rise in termperature [sic] continues.[11(p. 210)]

Her condition worsened, with weight loss and further deterioration of her mental status, but she received no more Prontosil. On August 5 she was transferred to the Neurological Institute of Columbia Medical Center, where she underwent temporal decompression to relieve the increased pressure in her head. A week later, unimproved with ongoing fever and now vomiting, she returned to Babies' Hospital.

Between August 21 and September 11, though unconscious, she received x-ray treatments to her head and spine because her father had read a report, again in the German medical literature, of its use in treating meningitis. Three months into her illness, on September 13, 1935, Katherine Woglom died.

The antibiotic had failed. Yet, it was a beginning—the first use of an antibiotic to treat a human infection in America, a small crack in the very large, until-then-closed door of medical therapeutics.

Alexander Ashley Weech, the physician who wrote the medical order to give Prontosil to Katherine Woglom, was born to Reverend Robert and Clara Ashley Weech in 1895. His father was a Methodist minister, and Ashley is said to have been reared in a home full of hard work, creativity, love, and compassion. Per family routine, Ashley and his brothers delivered a sermon each week after Sunday School on a topic of their choosing, an exercise that taught young Ashley proper diction and instilled in him a love of literature and the English language. Throughout his life, he was a stickler about words, syntax, and verbal clarity and demanded that his students and the authors of the papers he edited avoid dangling participles, ambiguous pronouns, and split infinitives. He quoted Chaucer regularly and insisted "children are 'reared' while laboratory rats are 'raised.' "[16(p. 229)]

He graduated from Johns Hopkins Medical School and then completed his pediatric training at the Harriet Lane Hospital in Baltimore. In accepting the American Pediatric Society's prestigious Howland Award (Figure 7.2), Weech recalled life as a pediatrician-in-training:

> During the first post-doctorate year, remuneration consisted of board and lodging shared with a companion house officer. Laundry was free, but I had to purchase the polish for my own shoes which custom decreed be kept in spotless white condition. During the second year, I enjoyed a room of my own plus a generous salary of

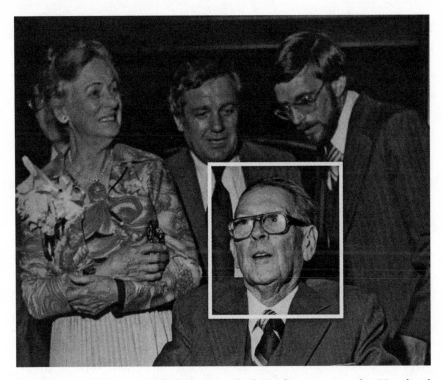

FIGURE 7.2 Dr. Alexander Ashley Weech (boxed) accepting the Howland Award, 1977, with his wife, Antonette-Hutton Weech.

From http://www.weech.net/ashley/John-Howland-Award_Dr-A-Ashley-Weech_and_Mrs-Antonette-Hutton-Weech_1977.jpg

$400 per annum. The comforts of life were at last coming my way. A third year and I was THE CHIEF! Now I merited room with private bath [*sic*]; pay for the year rocketed to $800. Since marital entanglement was absolutely taboo, subsistence was nominal and I lived the life of Croesus [wealthy king of ancient Lydia, known for vanity[9]]. On three occasions I sold blood "for transfusion" and for each sale the recompense was $50 per pint. I was rich, and soon became the possessor of a second-hand Model T Ford.[17(p. 232)]

After completing his pediatric training at Hopkins, Weech moved to China as pediatrician in chief at Peking Union Medical College. Two years later, he accepted an appointment at Babies' Hospital in New York, where he treated Katherine Woglom. Although his first use of an antibiotic in America is etched in the annals of pediatric infectious diseases history, Weech was not an infectious diseases doctor. Rather, he was a general pediatrician with the willingness, and courage, to try something new that might benefit his sick young patient. Further, his research focused on the metabolism of bilirubin (a breakdown product of red blood cells that is processed in the liver) rather than on bacteriology. In 1942, seven years after he treated Katherine with Prontosil, Weech relocated to the University of Cincinnati, where he was the chairman of pediatrics, and in 1975, he retired to the University of Florida in Gainesville.

Weech served as the editor of the *Journal of Diseases of Children* and as president of the American Pediatric Society. Besides being highly regarded as an outstanding teacher, researcher, clinician, and editor, he was renowned for his appreciation of the fine things of life, evidenced by his reputation as an eager fisherman and a dedicated wine connoisseur. Three months after receiving the Howland Award, he died in August 1977 from complications of heart disease.[16,18]

Weech's landmark role in delivering the first antibiotic used to treat a patient in America had, unfortunately, disappeared into the catacombs of time until Dr. Hugh Carithers, his friend from Jacksonville, Florida, wrote the historical essay of Katherine Woglom's illness and treatment in the *American Journal of Diseases of Childhood* in 1974, forty years after she was treated.[11]

Even though Prontosil failed to save Katherine Woglom's life and immune serum offered little to no benefit to patients with *H. influenzae* meningitis, physicians persisted in investigating the use of both sulfa drugs and influenzal immune serum to treat that infection. When Dr. Hattie Alexander at Columbia University in New York treated patients with *H. influenzae* meningitis with both influenzal immune serum made in rabbits and sulfa drugs, the survival rate was 74%,[19] considerably higher than that previously reported with no treatment, 2%—8%,[20,21] or with serum treatment alone, 6%–15%.[20,22] Dr. Josephine Neal from the New York City Health Department treated similar patients with influenzal immune serum made in horses plus a sulfa drug, and 48% survived.[23]

The sulfa drugs (several variations on Prontosil were used) proved somewhat effective in treating meningitis caused by bacteria other than

H. influenzae as well. Of 10 patients with meningococcal meningitis treated with sulfanilamide, 90% survived,[24] higher than the survival rates for patients treated with meningococcal immune serum alone (70%) or for those with no treatment (10%–30%).[25] This encouraged other scientists to try the sulfa drugs for many other types of infections. Patients with pneumococcal meningitis who were treated with sulfanilamide, however, had survival rates of only 20%–33%,[23,26] likely because pneumococci may be innately resistant to that drug. Although less than ideal, these results were far better than the dismal rates with only immune serum treatment—1 survivor among 631 patients with pneumococcal meningitis treated with pneumococcal immune serum.[27] Patients with hemolytic streptococcal (now called group A β-hemolytic streptococcal or *Streptococcus pyogenes*) meningitis had the best outcomes from sulfa therapy, with a survival rate of 80% compared to a rate of 5% with no treatment.[26]

The variability in meningitis survival rates after treatment with sulfa drugs was related to the use of different but related drugs, different doses, and different methods of administration (intravenous, intrathecal [directly into the spinal fluid], or oral), as well as different ages of the patients and varying duration of the infection prior to treatment. The antibiotic drugs weren't perfect, but they were a major breakthrough in treating patients with bacterial infections, including meningitis.

The world went crazy. Terrible infections of all kinds could now be cured or at least the patients had a better chance of surviving—not all of them, of course, but enough to generate considerable excitement. No longer did men need to lose their legs, or healthy newborns and women giving birth have to die, from infections. Sulfa was appropriately called the miracle drug, and its use exploded. In addition, the development of new sulfa drugs wasn't constrained by property rights due both to complicated patent issues involving German versus French law and to the fact that Prontosil is metabolized into two products, the red wine-colored dye and the colorless active ingredient sulfanilamide, whose previous patent as a chemical had expired. Thus, the race began among many pharmaceutical firms to bring these new antibiotics to market; by the mid-1940s. more than 5,000 sulfa drugs had been synthesized. Only a small number of those, however, actually made their way into medical practice.[28]

What do sulfa drugs do to the bacteria? Microbes, like all living organisms, require folic acid for growth, but, unlike humans who get folic acid in their diets, bacteria must manufacture it for themselves. Sulfa drugs inhibit the bacterial enzymatic pathway by which PABA (para-aminobenzoic acid) is transformed into folic acid.[29,30] Thus, sulfa drugs, in usual doses, starve the bacteria of the essential nutrient folic acid and thus prevent them from multiplying (i.e., the drugs are bacteriostatic) rather than killing them (i.e., the drugs are not bactericidal) as happened with immune serum treatment.

Sulfa drugs were actually the second class of antibiotics to be identified. The first were penicillins, members of the beta-lactam class of antimicrobial agents, which had been accidentally discovered by Dr. Alexander Fleming several years earlier and left to wallow in the dustbin of useless discoveries.

By 1928, Fleming, a Scottish physician who was a professor of bacteriology at St. Mary's Hospital Medical School, London, was an expert in the bacteria *Staphylococcus aureus* and was already famous for his discovery of lysozyme, an enzyme in tears, egg albumen, and nasal secretions that killed bacteria.[31] When he read a report showing that *S. aureus* could change its color from yellow-gold to white, change its texture from smooth to crenulated (scalloped), and change its character when clumping together from loosely sticky to very sticky,[32] Fleming decided to further explore the mechanisms that caused these phenomena.[33] In addition, he used *S. aureus* to facilitate the growth of *Bacillus influenzae* in his laboratory because the *S. aureus* produced, and released into the agar, the V growth factor (i.e., nicotinamide) necessary for *B. influenzae* to grow.[34]

Fleming, as many bacteriologists did, and still do, stored his bacteria on agar plates on his laboratory bench. When he returned from a month's vacation in Suffolk, the observant Fleming lifted the lid of one of the old plates of *S. aureus* and noted a patch of mold growing on the agar (Figure 7.3). Rather than snarling in frustration at the contaminated plate, he stared at the colonies of microorganisms and, according to one of Fleming's former students, said to his assistant, "That's funny."[33(p. 246)]

The "funny" thing Fleming saw was a ring around the mold, a halo in which *S. aureus* had barely grown. This suggested to him that the mold,

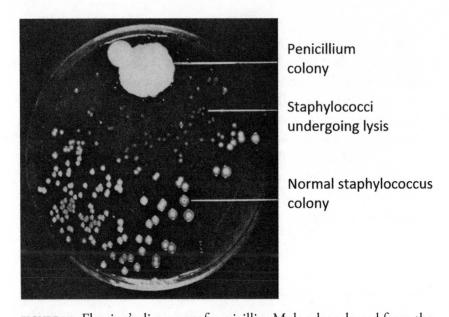

Penicillium colony

Staphylococci undergoing lysis

Normal staphylococcus colony

FIGURE 7.3 Fleming's discovery of penicillin. Molecules released from the colony of *Penicillium* mold killed the staphylococci surrounding it.

From Fleming A. On the Antibacterial Action of Cultures of a *Penicillium*, with Special Reference to Their Use in the Isolation of *B. influenzæ*. British Journal of Experimental Pathology. 1929;10(3):226–236.

which he originally thought was *Penicillium rubrum* and was later identified as *Penicillium notatum*, had somehow crippled the growth of the bacteria seated next to it.[35,36] Finally, after initially calling the toxic material emitted by the *Penicillium* "mould juice," Fleming settled on the name *penicillin* to reflect its origin from the mold. Although Fleming recognized the potential for mold extracts to treat patients with bacterial infections, he also knew that purifying the active ingredient from the mold would be very laborious, and he preferred to move on to other scientific endeavors. His discovery languished in the pages of the *British Journal of Experimental Pathology*.

In the course of his work with *Penicillium*, Fleming also recognized the capacity of the mold to improve the yield of *B. influenzae* from cultures of the respiratory tract. Most respiratory specimens contained other species of bacteria that could outgrow *B. influenzae* on agar, thus obscuring its presence. When Fleming cultured throat specimens on agar dishes that contained the mold extract, the unwanted bacteria didn't grow, but the *B. influenzae* flourished.[35] Thus was born the principle of "selective media," designer agar that contains antibiotics and thus suppresses the growth of undesirable microbes while preserving the growth of the bacteria under study.

While Alexander Fleming is widely credited with discovering penicillin, in truth the ability of the mold *Penicillium* to inhibit the growth of bacteria had been described 50 years earlier, within 2 years of each other, by two unheralded British scientists working independently.

In 1874, William Roberts devised a set of experiments to address a major scientific question of the day: Do bacteria arise de novo from sterile materials that are subjected to growth-promoting conditions, or do they arise from bacteria that had been imported onto the sterile materials? He crafted sterile glass chambers (Figure 7.4), in which he inserted various, presumably sterile, substances, such as egg albumen, blood, urine, and milk as well as juices from oranges, grapes, and tomatoes, and incubated them in "a warm place."[37]

About two-thirds of Roberts's samples remained sterile, while one-third grew bacteria, especially the samples that were difficult to keep sterile before planting them in the chambers. To him, this was proof that germs did not arise de novo by spontaneous generation from the test substances. In the article describing his experiments, the most interesting finding, however, was documented in a footnote addressing air contamination that occurred in some of the chambers (Figure 7.5). When the mold (also known as fungus) *Penicilium* [*sic*] *glaucum* grew in the chambers, he had difficulty getting bacteria to grow in them. As Roberts concluded, "It seemed, in fact, as if this fungus ... held in check the growth of *Bacteria*, with their attendant putrefactive changes."[37(p. 466)]

Two years later, when Dr. John Tyndall examined the possibility of spontaneous generation to explain putrefaction, he observed that bacteria failed to grow in cultures of turnip slices that had developed an overgrowth of "a beautiful tuft of mould," presumably *Penicillium*, whereas bacteria grew well in cultures free of the mold.[38]

Although Fleming (1929) had recognized the ability of penicillin to kill bacteria by 1930, it wasn't until after the sulfa drugs were found to effectively treat infections that the therapeutic potential of penicillin's

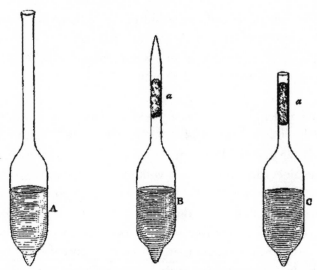

A. The bulb charged.   B. The bulb charged, plugged, and sealed ready for heating.   C. The bulb with its neck filed off, and set aside to see if it will germinate.   The figures are drawn about half the actual size.

FIGURE 7.4 Roberts's sterile tube experiment. An ordinary delivery pipette, with an oblong bulb capable of containing 30–50 mL, was sealed hermetically on the bottom (A). The materials of the experiment were placed into the bulb, and the neck of the bulb was plugged with cotton wool (B). The bulb was submerged in a can full of water, which was then boiled. After boiling, the bulb was cooled and filed off above the cotton wool plug to allow the materials access to filtered air (C). The bulb was maintained upright at the prescribed temperature and observed for bacterial growth.

From Roberts W. XII. Studies on Biogenesis. *Philosophical Transactions of the Royal Society of London*, 1874;164:460.

antibacterial effect was appreciated.[39] Because sulfa drugs were relatively useless in treating pneumococcal meningitis, a large collaborative study of penicillin for a variety of streptococcal infections, including those caused by pneumococci, was conducted. Of the 23 adults with pneumococcal meningitis treated with penicillin, 30% recovered.[40] The investigators had, however, used tiny doses of the drug. A subsequent study using massive doses given every 2 hours showed a survival rate of 62% in children.[41] This was much better than other treatments

Dr. SANDERSON'S experiments were planned on the supposition entertained by him that *Bacteria*-germs, while abundant in water, were almost absent from the air. In repeating some of his experiments, I failed in obtaining similar results. The air of the rooms wherein I worked was evidently highly charged with *Bacteria*-germs. In pursuing the inquiry, therefore, I sought to avoid air-contamination as sedulously as water-contamination‡.

The experiments which follow were all carried out on a plan which was, in principle, the same in every case. The materials of the experiment were enclosed in sterilized glass bulbs or tubes, which were plugged at one end with cotton-wool and hermetically sealed at the other. They were then set aside in a warm place to see if they would germinate.

The bulbs and tubes were prepared in the following manner :—They were first drawn out at the lower ends into capillary points (fig. 3, *b, b*) and sealed in the flame; the upper ends were plugged at *a, a* with cotton-wool.

* Annales de Chimie et de Physique, 1862, p. 66.
† Thirteenth Report of the Medical Officer of the Privy Council, p. 65.

‡ The avoidance of air-contamination is important for another reason. The air is admitted, by most observers, to be highly charged with fungoid germs, and the growth of fungi has appeared to me to be antagonistic to that of *Bacteria*, and *vice versâ*. I have repeatedly observed that liquids in which the *Penicillium glaucum* was growing luxuriantly could with difficulty be artificially infected with *Bacteria* ; it seemed, in fact, as if this fungus played the part of the plants in an aquarium, and held in check the growth of *Bacteria*, with their attendant putrefactive changes. On the other hand, the *Penicillium glaucum* seldom grows vigorously, if it grow at all, in liquids which are full of *Bacteria*.

FIGURE 7.5 Footnote that contains the original description of the bactericidal activity of *Penicillium glaucum* mold (the discovery of penicillin). From Roberts W. XII. Studies on Biogenesis. *Philosophical Transactions of the Royal Society of London,* 1874;164:457.

(i.e., sulfa or immune sera) for pneumococcal meningitis, but was still not optimal.

How did penicillin work? Penicillin-like, β-lactam-containing antibiotics interfere with the integrity of bacteria's envelope by inhibiting the enzymes that construct the bridges cross-linking the peptidoglycan molecules of the cell wall.[42] Basically, the penicillin molecule punches holes in the surface of the bacteria, their contents spill out, and the bacteria die. Thus, these drugs are bactericidal (killers) rather than bacteriostatic (growth inhibitors). Killer antibiotics are preferred to inhibitor antibiotics for treating meningitis.

Although penicillin successfully treated patients with pneumococcal and meningococcal meningitis, it didn't work well in treating *H. influenzae* meningitis. As Fleming observed when *H. influenzae* thrived in the presence of the *Penicillium* mold on culture plates, these bacteria are naturally resistant to penicillin. Sulfa drugs reduced deaths from influenzal meningitis somewhat, particularly when combined with influenzal immune serum, but Dr. Hattie Alexander, the pediatrician at Columbia University, thought she could do better. When she learned of the new antibiotic, streptomycin, she headed to her laboratory, conducted several experiments, and found that streptomycin killed all 22 of the *H. influenzae* meningitis strains she tested.[43] That was the proof she needed to use the drug for her patients.

The antibiotic streptomycin was discovered by Selman Waksman, a soil microbiologist at Rutgers University in New Jersey, who, in 1939, contemplated the fate of human bacterial pathogens. He noted bacteria that caused a number of human infections, including typhoid fever, dysentery, cholera, diphtheria, and tuberculosis, were not found in soil samples, even though sick people discharged their bacteria into the dirt with regularity. Waksman thus concluded that other bacteria in the soil must be antagonistic to the growth of human pathogens.[44] Unlike Fleming, who accidentally stumbled upon penicillin, Waksman and his graduate students, deliberately and methodically, began hunting for evidence of the antagonism they hypothesized.[45] They tested thousands of soil microbes and found about 20 that were antagonistic to bacterial growth. The bacteria *Actinomyces lavendulae*, for example, inhibited the growth of many gram-positive bacteria, but few gram negatives. His search further led him to the bacteria *Streptomyces griseus*, isolated from the dirt of a heavily manured field and from the throat of a chicken. This microbe killed a number of bacteria, including the human pathogens *Mycobacteria tuberculosis, Escherichia coli, S. aureus, Serratia marscesens*, and *Pseudomonas aeruginosa*.[46] The bactericidal substance in the *S. griseus* was named streptomycin in honor of the organism from which it was isolated.

When Alexander used streptomycin alone to treat children with either mild or moderate *H. influenzae* meningitis, 92% recovered, while more severe cases had lower recovery rates.[47] A larger study of sulfa plus streptomycin showed a survival rate of 97%[48] and assured physicians that antibiotics alone, without serum therapy, could successfully treat meningitis caused by *H. influenzae*.

The combination of a sulfa drug and streptomycin remained the standard treatment for influenzal meningitis until the 1950s,[49] when it was replaced with the antibiotic chloramphenicol.[50] Although *H. influenzae* bacteria are resistant to penicillin, they are usually sensitive to ampicillin, a cousin of penicillin. Limited, but encouraging, studies[51] led to the use of ampicillin to treat *H. influenzae* meningitis until the 1980s and the arrival of third-generation cephalosporins. These antibiotics, of the β-lactam class, are effective against all strains of *H. influenzae*, have relatively few side effects, and are reasonably easy to use.[52] Currently, ceftriaxone (or its relative cefotaxime) remain the standard treatment for both influenzal and meningococcal meningitis and, in combination with vancomycin, for pneumococcal meningitis, with survival rates of 95%, 92%, and 75%, respectively.[53]

In spite of the different kinds of bacteria that cause meningitis and the availability of various antibiotics to treat it, several basic principles of effective management for all common forms of bacterial meningitis have emerged from decades of research:

1. Rigorous attempts should be made to obtain cultures of the infecting bacteria from the spinal fluid (or the blood) of patients presenting with symptoms of meningitis so the exact cause of the infection can be determined and the bacteria can be assessed for antibiotic susceptibility (e.g., tests performed in the hospital microbiology laboratory to assess how well various antibiotics kill the bacteria). These test results are predictors (but not absolute proof) that specific antibiotics will effectively treat that patient's infection.
2. The patient's symptoms alone cannot predict the bacterial cause of meningitis as the symptoms associated with all bacterial causes overlap significantly. Further, Gram stains of the spinal fluid are useful guides to identifying the bacteria but may be difficult to interpret; antibiotic therapy should not be based solely on Gram stain results.
3. In general, the earlier in the course of the infection antibiotic treatment is delivered, the better the outcome.
4. Immediately on diagnosis of meningitis, empiric antibiotics (based on an educated guess from knowing the best therapy for common

bacteria that cause meningitis in similar patients) should be initiated until the patient's bacteria have been identified and their antimicrobial susceptibility patterns have been determined.

5. The ultimate, definitive antibiotic choice for an individual patient should be based on the measured antibiotic susceptibility of the bacteria infecting that patient.

6. Antibiotics that kill the bacteria (i.e., are bactericidal) are preferred over those that merely interfere with the growth of the bacteria (i.e., are bacteriostatic).

7. For effective therapy, adequate levels of the antibiotic must reach the site of the infection (i.e., the cerebrospinal fluid for meningitis). Irrespective of whether the antibiotic is given by mouth when appropriate or by vein, antibiotic levels in the blood are always higher, and sometimes significantly higher, than the corresponding levels in the spinal fluid. Thus, effective doses of antibiotics for meningitis must be high enough to ensure very high blood levels that will, in turn, provide adequate enough drug levels in the cerebrospinal fluid to treat the infection.

Over the past five decades, many animal experiments as well as clinical trials of antibiotics in humans treated for meningitis have defined the levels of antibiotics that are present in infected meninges and in the blood, thus informing the drug doses necessary to success-fully treat the infection.[54] As a result of these studies, most children with meningitis in America receive appropriate antibiotic treatment (the correct antibiotic and the correct dose for the correct duration of therapy), and their outcomes are much, much better than the dis-astrous outcomes of earlier eras.

References

1. Hippocrates. *On the Sacred Disease.* Adelaide, Australia: University of Adelaide; 2014.
2. Cullen W. *First Lines of the Practice of Physic,* (Vol. 1, 3rd ed.). Edinburgh: Creech; 1781.
3. Peacock M. Omens of Death. *Folk-lore.* 1890;8:377–378.
4. Sorapán de Rieros J, Sbarbi JM. *Medicina Española, Contenida en Proverbios Vulgares de Nuestra Lengua.* Madrid: Gómez Fuentenebro; 1876.

5. Foster GM. Relationships between Spanish and Spanish-American Folk Medicine. *Journal of American Folklore.* 1953;66(July–Sept):201–217.

6. Heister L, Davis C, Manby R, Innys W, Real Colegio de Cirugía de San Carlos (Madrid). *A General System of Surgery in Three Parts: Containing the Doctrine and Management.* London: printed for W. Innys in Paternester-Row, C. Davis against Grayt-Inn, J. Clark under the Royal Exchange, R. Manby and H. S. Cox on Ludgate-Hill, and J. Whiston in Fleet Street; 1750.

7. Kehoe MC. Fontanels: Issues and Setons in the Golden Age of Piracy. *The Pirate Surgeon's Journals: Tools and Procedures.* 2003. http://www.piratesurgeon.com/pages/surgeon_pages/fontanel1.html. Accessed December 2, 2016.

8. Dunglison R. *General Therapeutics, or Principles of Medical Practice, with Tables of the Chief Remedial Agents, etc.* Philadelphia: Carey, Lea, and Blanchard; 1836.

9. Simpson J, Weiner E. *Oxford English Dictionary.* Oxford, England: Oxford University Press; 1996.

10. Cooke J. *A Treatise on Nervous Disease. Vol. I on Apoplexy and Vol. II on Palsy and on Epilepsy.* London: Longman; 1820.

11. Carithers HA. The First Use of an Antibiotic in America. *American Journal of Diseases of Children.* 1974;128(2):207–211.

12. Domagk G. Ein Beitrag zur Chemotherapie der Bakteriellen Infektionen. *Deutsche medizinische Wochenschrift.* 1935;61(7):250–253.

13. Schreus HT. Chemotherapie des Erysipels und anderer Infektionen mit Prontosil. *Deutsche medizinische Wochenschrift.* 1935;61(7):255–256.

14. Anselm E. Unsere Erfahrungen mit Prontosil bei Puerperalfieber. *Deutsche medizinische Wochenschrift.* 1935;61(7):264.

15. Klee P, Romer H. Prontosil bei Streptokokken-enkrankungen. *Deutsche medizinische Wochenschrift.* 1935;61(7):255–256.

16. Ayoub EM. Introduction of Dr. A. Ashley Weech for the John Howland Award: From the American Pediatric Society, April 27, 1977, San Francisco, California. *Pediatric Research.* 1978;12(3):229–231.

17. Weech AA. John Howland Award Acceptance Address: From the American Pediatric Society, April 27, 1977, San Francisco, California. *Pediatric Research.* 1978;12(3):232–234.

18. Forbes GB. Alexander Ashley Weech, MD. *American Journal of Diseases of Children.* 1977;131(10):1075–1075.

19. Alexander HE, Ellis C, Leidy G. Treatment of Type-Specific *Hemophilus influenzae* Infections in Infancy and Childhood. *The Journal of Pediatrics.* 1942;20(6):673–698.

20. Fothergill LRD. *Hemophilus influenzae* (Pfeiffer Bacillus) Meningitis and Its Specific Treatment. *New England Journal of Medicine.* 1937;216(14):587–590.

21. Rivers TM. Influenzal Meningitis. *American Journal of Diseases of Children.* 1922;24(2):102–124.

22. Pittman M. The Action of Type-Specific Hemophilus Influenzae Antiserum. *The Journal of Experimental Medicine.* 1933;58(6):683–706.

23. Neal JB, Appelbaum E, Jackson HW. Sulfapyridine and Its Sodium Salt: In the Treatment of Meningitis Due to the *Pneumococcus* and *Haemophilus influenzae. Journal of the American Medical Association.* 1940;115(24):2055–2058.

24. Schwentker FF, Gelman S, Long PH. The Treatment of Meningococcic Meningitis with Sulfanilamide: Preliminary Report. *Journal of the American Medical Association.* 1937;108(17):1407–1408.

25. Flexner S. The Results of the Serum Treatment in Thirteen Hundred Cases of Epidemic Meningitis. *The Journal of Experimental Medicine.* 1913;17(5):553–576.

26. Neal JB. The Treatment of Acute Infections of the Central Nervous System with Sulfanilamide. *Journal of the American Medical Association.* 1938;111(15):1353–1356.

27. Waring GW, Weinstein L. The Treatment of Pneumococcal Meningitis. *The American Journal of Medicine.* 1948;5(3):402–418.

28. Lesch JE. *The First Miracle Drugs: How the Sulfa Drugs Transformed Medicine.* Oxford, England: Oxford University Press; 2007.

29. Smith CL, Powell KR. Review of the Sulfonamides and Trimethoprim. *Pediatrics in Review.* 2000;21(11):368–371.

30. Henry RJ. The Mode of Action of Sulfonamides. *Bacteriological Reviews.* 1943;7(4):175–262.

31. Fleming A. On a Remarkable Bacteriolytic Element Found in Tissues and Secretions. *Proceedings of the Royal Society of London.* 1922;93:301–317.

32. Bigger JW, Boland CR, O'Meara RAQ. Variant Colonies of *Staphylococcus aureus. The Journal of Pathology and Bacteriology.* 1927;30(2):261–269.

33. Diggins F. The True History of the Discovery of Penicillin by Alexander Fleming. *Biomedical Scientist.* 2003;March:246–249.

34. Grassberger R. Beiträge zur Bakteriologie der Influenza. *Zeitschrift für Hygiene und Infektionskrankheiten.* 1897;25(3):453–476.

35. Fleming A. On the Antibacterial Action of Cultures of a Penicillium, with Special Reference to Their Use in the Isolation of *B. influenzæ. British Journal of Experimental Pathology.* 1929;10(3):226–236.

36. Fleming A. Penicillin. Nobel Prize Lecture. 1945. https://www.nobelprize. org/prizes/medicine/1945/fleming/lecture/. Accessed January 2, 2017.

37. Roberts W. Studies on Biogenesis. *Philosophical Transactions of the Royal Society of London.* 1874;164:457–477.

38. Tyndall J. The Optical Deportment of the Atmosphere in Relation to the Phenomena of Putrefaction and Infection. *Philosophical Transactions of the Royal Society of London.* 1876;166:27–74.

39. Chain E, Florey HW, Gardner AD, et al. Penicillin as a Chemotherapeutic Agent. *The Lancet.* 1940;236(6104):226–228.

40. Keefer CS, Blake FG, Marshall E, et al. Penicillin in the Treatment of Infections: A Report of 500 Cases. *Journal of the American Medical Association.* 1943;122(18):1217–1224.

41. Dowling HF, Sweet LK, Robinson JA, Zellers WA, Hirsh HL. The Treatment of Pneumococcic Meningitis with Massive Doses of Systemic Penicillin. *American Journal of the Medical Sciences.* 1949;217(2):149–156.

42. Doi Y, Chambers HF. Penicillins and β-Lactamase Inhibitors. In: Bennett JE, Dolin R, Blaser MJ, eds. *Mandell, Douglas, and Bennett's Principles and Practice of Infectious Diseases.* Philadelphia: Elsevier-Saunders; 2014:263–277.

43. Alexander HE, Leidy G. Influence of Streptomycin on Type b *Haemophilus influenzae. Science.* 1946;104(2692):101–102.

44. Waksman SA, Woodruff HB. The Soil as a Source of Microorganisms Antagonistic to Disease-Producing Bacteria. *Journal of Bacteriology.* 1940;40(4):581–600.

45. Ginsberg J. Selman Waksman and Antibiotics. American Chemical Society National Historic Chemical Landmarks. 2005. http://www.acs.org/content/acs/en/education/whatischemistry/landmarks/selmanwaksman.html. Accessed February 21, 2017.

46. Schatz A, Bugie E, Waksman SA. Streptomycin, a Substance Exhibiting Antibiotic Activity Against Gram-Positive and Gram-Negative Bacteria. *Proceedings of the Society for Experimental Biology and Medicine.* 1944;55(1):66–69.

47. Alexander HE, Leidy G, Rake G, Donovick R. *Hemophilus influenzae* Meningitis Treated with Streptomycin. *Journal of the American Medical Association.* 1946;132(8):434–440.

48. Appelbaum E, Nelson J. Streptomycin in the Treatment of Influenzal Meningitis: A Study of Ninety Cases, with 96.6% Recovery. *Journal of the American Medical Association.* 1950;143(8):715–717.

49. Turk DC, May JR. Hemophilus influenzae: *Its Clinical Importance.* London: English Universities Press; 1967.

50. Haggerty RJ, Ziai M. Acute Bacterial Meningitis in Children: A Controlled Study of Antimicrobial Therapy, with Particular Reference to Combinations of Antibiotics. *Pediatrics.* 1960;25(5):742–747.

51. Thrupp LD, Leedom JM, Ivler D, et al. *H. Influenzæ* Meningitis: A Controlled Study of Treatment with Ampicillin. *Postgraduate Medical Journal.* 1964;40(Suppl.):119–125.

52. Stutman HR, Marks MI. Bacterial Meningitis in Children: Diagnosis and Therapy: A Review of Recent Developments. *Clinical Pediatrics.* 1987;26(9):431–438.

53. Swartz MN. Bacterial Meningitis—A View of the Past 90 Years. *New England Journal of Medicine.* 2004;351(18):1826–1828.

54. McCracken GH. Management of Bacterial Meningitis: Current Status and Future Prospects. *The American Journal of Medicine.* 1984;76(5):215–223.

8

Microbes and Genetics

DAISIES ARE DAISIES, AND beagles are beagles. Likewise, ladybugs are ladybugs, and people are people. The beautiful, intriguing, beguiling characteristics that make us who we are don't appear out of nowhere. Most are inherited from our parents: Redheads beget redheads. Tall pea plants beget tall pea plants. And yet, daisies are different; not all are exactly alike. Same for beagles, redheads, tall pea plants, and ladybugs. The same holds for people and, of course, bacteria.

Dr. Margaret Pittman first identified a major factor in which *Haemophilus. influenzae* strains are different from one other—their bacterial capsules, those polysaccharide overcoats that are woven from complex sugars and surround the bacterial cell.[1] The bacteria she studied have one of six distinct kinds of capsules (types a–f) as defined by their ability to agglutinate (clump) when mixed with capsule-specific immune sera, or they have no capsule. Further, type a strains beget type a strains, type b strains beget type b strains, and so forth. Pittman also showed, however, that *H. influenzae* Smooth strains (those with a slimy capsule) may lose their capsules and become Rough—their surfaces appear raggedy because they have no slimy capsule—when the bacteria are grown, generation after generation, on agar. Smooth thus beget Smooth, except that sometimes they beget Rough. The opposite effect, Rough spawning Smooth strains, however, didn't happen even when bacteria were repeatedly passed on agar for many, many generations. Pittman's Rough strains had lost the sugar coating that had

Continual Raving: A History of Meningitis and the People Who Conquered It. Janet R Gilsdorf, Oxford University Press (2020). © Oxford University Press.
DOI: 10.1093/oso/9780190677312.001.0001

made them Smooth, but, once lost, they couldn't regain it. Why? What master regulator of their inheritance explained that? If it wasn't about money, it must have had something to do with their genes.

Fred Griffith, a British physician and bacteriologist, doggedly pursued his passion for the epidemiology of lung infections in the early 1920s while working at the Ministry of Health Laboratory in London. This government facility, while old and rundown, was regarded by British doctors as the model for excellent bacteriology service.[2] There Griffith labored side by side with W. McDonald Scott, a pathologist, in cramped quarters on the third floor of Dudley House at 36 Endell Street (Figure 8.1). The bottom two floors of Dudley House held the neighborhood post office. The building had originally been built in 1878 by brothers William A. and Arthur Beresford Pite as an infirmary for the St. Giles-in-the-Fields parish workhouse, which was essentially a poorhouse.[3]

Visiting scientists were appalled by the limited space and primitive conditions of this outstanding national laboratory, calling it a disgrace from "a great department of a wealthy country."[4(p. 2)] The laboratory consisted of one small office, the actual laboratory, and a media kitchen where two technicians prepared the broths and agar plates for the microbiologic experiments. Griffith and Scott's ability to produce good science in such an overcrowded place was credited to their capacity to "do more with a kerosene tin and primus stove than most men could do with a palace."[5(p. 588)]

Even Parliament became aware of the miserable conditions at Dudley House when Sir J. Remnant notified the financial secretary of the Treasury

> that the [post office] lavatory accommodation is defective and inadequate, that much of the lighting is bad, that the heating is imperfect, that the ventilation requires considerable attention, and that, owing to the joint operation of many punching machines and tabulators in a crowded room, many of the female staff suffer from nerves. In view of the complaints which exist with regard to practically every room in the building, [will he] cause a thorough investigation to be made, with a view to removing the disadvantages under which the staff labour?

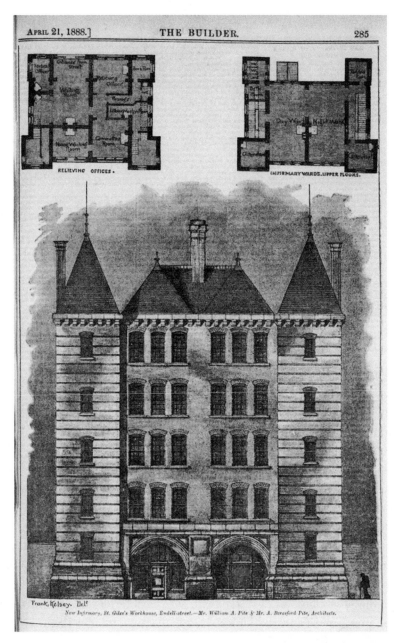

RELIEVING OFFICES.

INFIRMARY WARDS. UPPER FLOORS.

Frank. Kelsey. Del.

New Infirmary, St. Giles's Workhouse, Endell-street.—Mr. William A. Pite & Mr. A. Beresford Pite, Architects.

FIGURE 8.1 Drawing of the St. Giles-in-the-Fields workhouse/infirmary that later became Dudley House where Fred Griffith's laboratory was located.

From Beresford Pite W, Beresford Pite A. New Infirmary, St. Gile's Workhouse, Endell Street. *The Builder.* 1888;54:285.

Mr. Graham responded, "My attention has not previously been drawn to this matter, and I am having inquiries made."[6]

Six years later, things were no better. Again, a constituent, Mr. W. J. Brown, appealed to Parliament. He asked the postmaster general

> whether he is aware of the outbreak of boils and carbuncles among the staff of the mechanical transport section of the Post Office stores housed in the old workhouse in Endell Street; whether he is aware that the accommodation in this building is infested with mice, which are themselves affected with skin diseases; whether he is aware that in the same building there is a bacteriology laboratory; and whether he will either remove his staff from the building or take steps to remove the vermin and the bacteria?[7]

Mr. Lees-Smith was aware of the boils and carbuncles and, after a medical inspection, he was advised, "that there is no connection between this outbreak and the proximity of a bacteriology laboratory or the presence of mice in the building. ... Urgent measures are being taken to exterminate the mice."

A Mr. McQuisten suggested, "Could not the Postmaster-General get a number of cats to inflict capital punishment on the mice?"[7] This miserable, infested building was where Griffith and Scott conducted their magnificent work.

Frederick Griffith was born in Eccleston in Lancashire, England, to Joseph Griffith (a farmer) and his wife, Emily Louise, nee Hackett. The date of Fred's birth has been cited as either 1877 or 1879, but based on birth and census records from Lancashire, 1877 is likely correct.[8,9] There were four Griffith sons in their household in the village of Hale: Thomas, who became a civil engineer; Arthur Stanley and Frederick, who both became physicians; and George, who became a farmer like their father. Fred graduated from the University of Liverpool Medical School and completed a fellowship in pathology in Liverpool.[5] Early in his professional career, he worked with his brother Stanley, a prominent physician and medical scientist, for the Royal Commission on tuberculosis.

Fred strongly believed "that a proper understanding of epidemiologic problems could come only from more detailed and discriminating knowledge of infectious bacterial species, and of the nature of bacterial virulence and variation."[10](p. 385) At that time, bacteria were thought to be fixed in character and their physical features were expected to remain the same over many generations. Griffith was interested in, and probably frustrated by, the fact that pneumococci, like *H. influenzae*, didn't remain the same, but, rather, flipped, seemingly haphazardly, from Smooth to Rough forms while growing on agar.[11] They were like spirits he just couldn't tame.

Griffith was a loner, a shy and aloof man who was difficult to get to know.[4] He was devoted to his work to the exclusion of most other activities, except for skiing during the winter in the Alps, taking his dog, Bobby, on walks (Figure 8.2), and relaxing in a cottage he had built

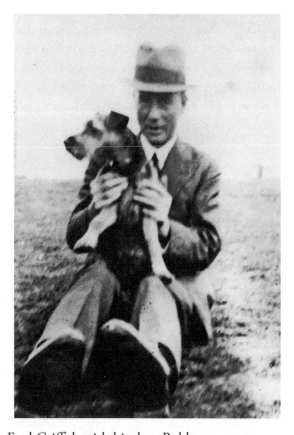

FIGURE 8.2 Fred Griffith with his dog, Bobby.

From the National Library of Medicine. https://profiles.nlm.nih.gov/ps/retrieve/ResourceMetadata/CCAABN.

on the Sussex Downs.[5] He rarely attended scientific meetings, and he nervously and reluctantly gave one, and only one, rather boring scientific presentation during his entire professional life; he reportedly had to be almost forced into a taxi to get to that meeting, the 1936 London International Microbiology Congress.[11]

Griffith was immensely hard working, neurotically careful, and scrupulously honest in his research, and, while his scientific papers were well respected, they were few in number. He took a long time to publish his work, as he chronically questioned his results, repeated the experiments many times, and used many, many controls. Regarding the slow pace of his publications, he said, "Almighty God is in no hurry—why should I be?"[5(p. 588)] His papers methodically described the experiments and presented them in a well-organized, logical form that permitted the reader to follow his thinking during each step in the process. In writing about pneumococci, he ascribed intention to them and spoke of the microbes as if they were his bacterial buddies, "By assuming the R [Rough] form, the pneumococcus has admitted defeat"[12(p. 156)] and "while the R form may be the final stage in the struggle of the bacterium to preserve its individuality."[12(p. 157)]

In the course of his studies of lung infections, Griffith collected pneumococcal strains from patients with pneumonia and identified four different capsular types, I–IV. The questions that drove his subsequent experiments were (1) "Do serological [capsule] types represent stages in the normal life history of a bacterium or are they the response on the part of the bacterium to changes in the immunological state of the animal host?"[12(p. 147)] and (2) Are the influences that promote different serological types of bacteria at play because of altered environments in which they are grown? Basically, he wondered if the various pneumococcal capsule types represented developmental stages of the bacteria, or if they changed because of an immunologic influence from the infected patient or because of an unknown environmental influence. He set about to answer these questions by injecting various combinations of live and dead pneumococci under the skin of mice.[12]

As a control for his experiments on pneumococcal capsules, he injected a mixture of dead, Smooth forms of type I pneumococci and alive, Rough forms of type II pneumococci into the mice, and the animals became sick. To Griffith's surprise, cultures of the heart's blood from the ill mice grew live, Smooth type I organisms in spite of the fact that the live bacteria he had injected were Rough type II. It looked as if something from the dead, type I strains he had included in the injections had been incorporated into the alive type II strains, turning them into living type I strains (Figure 8.3). He found these results hard to believe and, in his compulsive way, repeated the experiments many times, using multiple combinations of live and dead, Rough and Smooth, types I–IV strains. The conclusions from his experiments were always the same: Dead, Smooth pneumococci were able to "transform"—his word—live, Rough pneumococci into live Smooth pneumococci.[12]

Griffith had no idea how the process he called transformation actually worked, and he was not aware of the enormous impact his observations would ultimately have on the field of bacteriology and, indeed, on all of science. In fact, in the extremely comprehensive paper describing those experiments—the only paper he published on the topic—his transformation results were wedged among many other, more mundane, epidemiologic details of pneumococcal pneumonia and the findings of pneumococcal virulence in mice.[12] While his observations were very accurate, his ultimate conclusions about some aspects of the

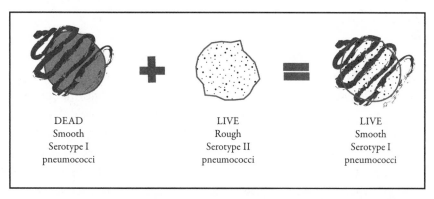

FIGURE 8.3 Griffith's transformation experiments with dead and live pneumococci. Type I capsule genes from dead bacteria are transformed into live, Rough, nonencapsulated type II pneumococci, and the resulting live bacteria have type I capsule.

Drawing by the author.

results—that transformation wasn't abrupt but rather was the result of evolution, with the Rough form acting as an intermediary between two types of Smooth forms—were very wrong.[11] He was also wrong in thinking that the capsule itself, facilitated by a protein of some sort, mediated the transformation. After he completed those pneumococcal studies, he moved on to other bacteria.

Griffith's work remained unheralded, and largely unnoticed, although other scientists confirmed that bacterial transformation could occur in test tubes as well as in mice,[13] a feat Griffith had been unable to accomplish. In addition, subsequent studies by other scientists gradually refined the nature of the transforming material, showing it to be an active agent present in filtered extracts that lacked all formed elements and were free of cellular debris.[14]

After publishing his paper on the transformation of the pneumococcal capsule from a Smooth strain to a Rough strain, which, unbeknown to him, was the first clue to understanding the movement of genetic traits from one bacterium to another, Griffith continued to quietly, meticulously labor in the Ministry of Health laboratory on Endell Street, year after year, with McDonald Scott. On the night of April 17, 1941, they were together at Griffith's flat when it rained fire, plaster from the walls, and bricks from the chimney. The building had been hit by a German bomb during the London Blitz. Both Griffith and Scott and Griffith's housekeeper perished in the attack.[15]

In the 1940s, the leading scientist studying pneumococci was Oswald Avery at the Rockefeller Institute. Initially, and privately, Avery largely discounted Griffith's results with pneumococcal transformation and thought the findings were explained by inadequate controls.[4] Griffith would have been horrified to learn of Avery's opinion, as he obsessed over the quality of his experiments and used an endless number of controls. Further, he greatly admired Avery from afar. Ultimately, after Avery's associates confirmed the ability of dead Smooth pneumococci to transform living Rough strains into Smooth strains, Avery sought to isolate the active principle in bacteria responsible for the transformation and to define its chemical composition. His experiments showed that a bacterial fraction isolated from a type III pneumococcal strain, which was able to transform a Rough type II strain into a Smooth type

III strain, was composed of deoxyribonucleic acid, or DNA, a complex molecule of sugars and nucleic acids. He called the fraction the "transforming principle,"[16] appropriating Griffith's word to name the agent of transformation. In a letter to his brother, Roy, also a scientist, Avery wrote that the transforming principle "is in all probability DNA: who could have guessed it?"[11(p. 11)]

Several years after Avery and his colleagues published their landmark paper (for which the authors received the Nobel Prize), Stephen Zaminof and Erwin Chargaff noted that DNA isolated from yeast was different from that of pancreatic cells, and that these differences were "in harmony with the hypothesis connecting nucleic acids with the transmission of hereditary characteristics."[17(p. 737)] Further, that same year Harriett Taylor, a colleague of Avery's, showed that the transforming principles, indeed, were responsible for heredity in bacteria and wrote, "It appears justified to visualize the transforming principle much as the geneticist pictures genes."[18(p. 400)] Five years later, James Watson and Francis Crick determined the actual chemical structure of DNA and proposed the template mechanism by which DNA duplicates itself,[19] thus firmly defining the molecules that convey heredity. DNA (Figure 8.4), indeed, was destiny.

The concept of heredity was well known even in 400 BCE at the time of Hippocrates, whose theory of inheritance suggested that "inherited qualities, in some way or other, must have been transmitted to the new individual from different parts of the [bodies of the] father and the mother."[20] In addition, Charles Darwin used the word *genetic* as a biologic term to connote an adjectival form of the word *origin*. He wrote, "It is incredible that the descendants of two organisms, which had originally differed in a marked manner, should ever afterwards converge so closely as to lead to a near approach to identity throughout their whole organisation."[21,22]

A decade later, in 1911, Wilhelm Johannsen, a plant physiologist from the University of Copenhagen, addressed the American Society of Naturalists and riffed on the need for words to express the concept of heredity, which he defined as "the transmission of the parent's (or ancestor's) *personal qualities* to the progeny." Further, he considered those personal qualities to be "*the reactions of the gametes* [egg and

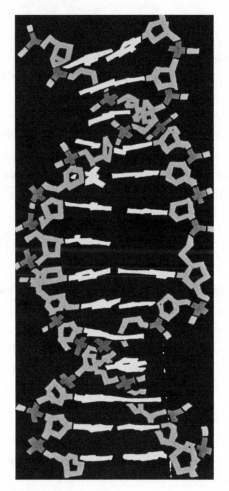

FIGURE 8.4 Schematic of DNA.

From the National Library of Medicine. https://collections.nlm.nih.gov/catalog/ nlm:nlmuid-101456157-img.

sperm cells] joining to form a zygote [fertilized egg that becomes an embryo]."[23(p. 129)] In his speech, Johannsen stated that, "Language is not only our servant when we wish to express—or even to conceal—our thoughts, but that it may also be our master, overpowering us by means of the notions attached to the current words."[23(p. 132)]

Johannsen then proposed the addition of the terms *gene* and *genotype* to the genetic lexicon. He considered the term *gene* to be "nothing but a very applicable little word, easily combined with others, and hence it may be useful as an expression for the 'unit-factors,' 'elements,' or 'allelomorphs' in the gametes," and a *genotype* to be "the sum total of all the genes in the gamete or in a zygote."[23(p. 132)] In the same lecture, he proposed the words *phenotype* (the totality of observable characteristics) and *biotype* (the shared genetic composition of clusters of subspecies having similar characteristics). At that time, although the chemical nature of genes wasn't known, their heritability action had long been recognized. Not until the original work of Griffith[12] and the clarifying work of Avery[16] were the basic agents of inheritance—transforming principles, or DNA—identified.

Avery had very convincingly demonstrated that transforming principles (DNAs) of pneumococci carried information that controlled the character of those bacteria, but it wasn't clear if the phenomenon was limited to pneumococci or if it was present in other bacteria. Studies in *Escherichia coli* and *Shigella* had been inconclusive.[24] Dr. Hattie Alexander, the pediatrician at Babies' Hospital in New York who pioneered the use of antibiotics and influenzal immune serum to treat influenzal meningitis, wondered if *H. influenzae* also had the transforming principle. These bacteria, after all, were very different from pneumococci, which are coccoid (round balls) and have a positive Gram stain, while *H. influenzae* bacteria are short rods and gram negative. Could *H. influenzae*, like pneumococci, also exchange genetic traits through transformation?

Along with her laboratory assistant, Grace Leidy, Alexander prepared DNA from a type b Smooth *H. influenzae* strain and crude transforming principles from each of the other types (a, c–f) and mixed them with living Rough bacteria derived, by loss of the capsule, from each type. All of the strains except type f underwent transformation. It was, however, spotty since not every Rough strain could be transformed into Smooth strains of every type. Stain Rd (a Rough variant of a type d *H. influenzae* strain) was the winner, as it could be successfully transformed into Smooth variants of all six types (Table 8.1).[25] (Note: Remember strain Rd, as it is discussed in further chapters.) Further, *H. influenzae* was easier to transform than pneumococci. The process in pneumococci required both a special environment beyond ordinary growth conditions and time to sensitize the bacterial cells to be transformed.

TABLE 8.1 Transformation of *H. influenzae* capsule genes from smooth strains (types a–f) to rough strains

Rough (R) mutants	Result of exposure of the rough *H. influenzae* mutants to transforming principles (TP) from the 6 types					
	TP type a	TP type b	TP Type c	TP type d	TP type e	TP type f
R type a	S type a	o	o	o	o	o
R type b	S type a	S type b	S type c	S type d	o	o
R type c	o	o	o	o	o	o
R type d	S type a	S type b	S type c	S type d	S type e	S type f
R type e	o	o	o	o	o	o
R type f	o	o	o	o	o	o

R = rough bacteria (no capsule)
S = smooth bacteria (has a capsule)

Adapted from Hattie Alexander and Grace Leidy, Determination of Inherited Traits of H. influenzae by Desoxyribonucleic Acid Fractions Isolated from Type-Specific Cells, J Exp Med 1951; 93: 345–359.

Thus, in the laboratory, the transforming principle (i.e., DNA) from Smooth strains of every *H. influenzae* capsule type could convert (or transform) Rough strains that had lost their capsules into Smooth strains, although such a conversion didn't occur naturally among Rough strains—Rough strains didn't beget Smooth strains when passed in pure culture for many generations. Alexander and Leidy showed that Rough meningococci could also be transformed to Smooth forms by exposure to the DNA of Smooth strains.[26] In short, the three kinds of bacteria that caused most of the cases of meningitis in children, *H. influenzae*, pneumococci, and meningococci, could be made to acquire new characteristics, such as capsule type, by exposing them to DNA, or transforming principle, from a strain with the desired characteristic, such as a specific capsule. A new day in bacteriology, one in which their genetic workings could be explored, had dawned.

References

1. Pittman M. The Action of Type-Specific *Hemophilus influenzae* Antiserum. *The Journal of Experimental Medicine.* 1933;58(6):683–706.
2. Wilson GS. The Public Health Laboratory Service: Origin and Development of Public Health Laboratories. *The British Medical Journal.* 1948;1(4553):677–682.

3. Higginbotham P. St. Giles-in-the-Fields and St. George Bloomsbury, Middlesex, London. The Workhouse: The Story of an Institution. 2017. http://www.workhouses.org.uk/StGiles/. Accessed July 31, 2017.

4. Downie AW. Pneumococcal Transformation—A Backward View, Fourth Griffith Memorial Lecture. *Microbiology.* 1972;73(1):1–11.

5. Wright HD. Fredrick Griffith. *The Lancet.* 1941;237(6140):588–589.

6. House of Commons. Customs Statistics Office, Endell Street. Government Departments. 1924;177:c346W. https://api.parliament.uk/historic-hansard/written-answers/1924/oct/02/customs-statistics-office-endell-street. Accessed June 4, 2017.

7. House of Commons. Stores, Endell Street (Accommodation). 1930;236:1907–1908. https://api.parliament.uk/historic-hansard/commons/1930/mar/18/stores-endell-street-accommodation. Accessed June 4, 2017.

8. Find My Past. Results for England and Wales Births 1837–2006. 2016. http://search.findmypast.com/results/world-records/england-and-wales-births-1837-2006?firstname=fredrick&firstname_variants=true&lastname=griffith&_page=2. Accessed December 30, 2016.

9. Ancestry.com. Frederick Griffith. http://person.ancestry.com/tree/10404752/person/140046403895/facts. Accessed December 30, 2016.

10. Hayes W. Genetic Transformation: A Retrospective Appreciation. *Journal of General Microbiology.* 1966;45:385–397.

11. Pollack MR. The Discovery of DNA: An Ironic Tale of Chance, Prejudice and Insight. *Journal of General Microbiology.* 1970;63:1–20.

12. Griffith F. The Significance of Pneumococcal Types. *Journal of Hygiene.* 1928;27(2):113–159.

13. Dawson MH, Sia RHP. In Vitro Transformation of Pneumococcal Types. *Journal of Experimental Medicine.* 1931;54(5):681–699.

14. Alloway JL. The Transformation In Vitro of R Pneumococci into S Forms of Different Specific Types by the Use of Filtered Pneumococcus Extracts. *The Journal of Experimental Medicine.* 1932;55(1):91–99.

15. Méthot P-O. Bacterial Transformation and the Origins of Epidemics in the Interwar Period: The Epidemiological Significance of Fred Griffith's "Transforming Experiment." *Journal of the History of Biology.* 2016;49(2):311–358.

16. Avery OT, MacLeod CM, McCarty M. Studies on the Chemical Nature of the Substance Inducing Transformation of Pneumococcal Types. *Journal of Experimental Medicine.* 1944;79(2):137–158.

17. Zamenhof S, Chargaff E. Studies on the Desoxypentose Nuclease of Yeast and Its Specific Cellular Regulation. *Journal of Biological Chemistry.* 1949;180(2):727–740.

18. Taylor HE. Additive Effects of Certain Transforming Agents from Some Variants of Pneumococcus. *The Journal of Experimental Medicine.* 1949;89(4):399–424.

19. Watson JD, Crick FHC. Genetical Implications of the Structure of Deoxyribonucleic Acid. *Nature.* 1953;171(4361):964–967.

20. Henschen F. The Nobel Prize in Physiology or Medicine 1933: Presentation Speech. 1933. http://www.nobelprize.org/nobel_prizes/medicine/laureates/1933/press.html. Accessed December 11, 2016.

21. Darwin C. *The Origin of Species by Means of Natural Selection.* New York: Crowell; 1899.

22. Simpson J, Weiner E. *Oxford English Dictionary.* Oxford, England: Oxford University Press; 1996.

23. Johannsen W. The Genotype Conception of Heredity. *The American Naturalist.* 1911;45(531):129–159.

24. Weil AJ, Binder M. Experimental Type Transformation of *Shigella paradysenteriae* (Flexner). *Experimental Biology and Medicine.* 1947;66(2):349–352.

25. Alexander HE, Leidy G. Transformation Type Specificity of *H. influenzae. Proceedings of the Society for Experimental Biology and Medicine.* 1950;73(3):485–487.

26. Alexander HE, Redman W. Transformation of Type Specificity of Meningococci. *The Journal of Experimental Medicine.* 1953;97(6):797–806.

9

Antibiotics: Sometimes They Fail

IMAGINE A WORLD IN which all bacteria that cause meningitis are resistant to every antibiotic in our therapeutic armamentarium, a time
when doctors have no drugs to treat this deadly infection, a return to
the days before Alexander Fleming discovered penicillin and Gerhard
Domagk discovered sulfa. We'd be back to the era of very bad outcomes
in children with meningitis: Most would die, and the rare survivors
would be deaf, blind, or developmentally delayed or have cerebral palsy.

The advent of antibiotics revolutionized the practice of medicine. In
a relatively short time after their introduction, infections treated with
these drugs sometimes yielded complete recovery where chronic dis-
ability or death had previously prevailed. In the intervening 80 years,
antibiotics have prevented many millions of deaths from infections
and contributed to the increased human life span. Doctors use them
daily to treat otitis media, cellulitis, sinusitis, urinary tract infections,
or pneumonia and to save the lives of countless children with terrible
infections, such as endocarditis, septicemia, necrotizing cellulitis, and
meningitis. Not only do antibiotics, if given early enough, keep patients
with meningitis from dying, but also, as a result of effective treatment,
many of these patients now recover with little or no neurologic damage.

The miracle of antibiotics presented a promise that all infectious diseases could be cured, forever. In fact, the former surgeon general of
the United States, Dr. William H. Stewart, has been widely reported
to have claimed, in either 1967 or 1969, "It's time to close the book on
infectious diseases, and declare the war against pestilence won." His

Continual Raving: A History of Meningitis and the People Who Conquered It. Janet
R Gilsdorf, Oxford University Press (2020). © Oxford University Press.
DOI: 10.1093/oso/9780190677312.001.0001

statement, however, appears to be an urban myth. In spite of diligent searches, Brad Spellberg and Bonnie Taylor-Blake could find no documentation that Stewart ever uttered those words.[1] Only a fool—and Stewart was no fool—would think eliminating all infections, for all time, could be possible.

In her quest to find the optimal therapy for her patients with *Haemophilus influenzae* meningitis, Hattie Alexander, the pediatrician at Columbia University who studied influenzal immune serum, was immediately drawn to the experiments of Albert Schatz and colleagues when they identified a new drug, streptomycin, that had bactericidal activity against a number of bacteria, including *Escherichia coli*, *Staphylococcus aureus*, *Pseudomonas aeruginosa*, and *Aeromonas aerogenes*.[2] They hadn't, however, studied *H. influenzae* in those early reports.

So, Alexander headed to her laboratory to devise a method to predict if streptomycin might treat infections caused by *H. influenzae*. She gathered *H. influenzae* strains from patients before they received treatment; mixed a standard quantity of those bacteria (the number of organisms contained in a 2-mm wire loop) with various concentrations of streptomycin; and cultured the resultant brew on agar plates. When she counted the surviving bacteria, she discovered that fewer than 10 units of the antibiotic prevented visible growth of the *H. influenzae*. She called this effect the "minimal effective concentration" of streptomycin necessary to impede the bacteria's growth.[3] Although not well recognized in the medical literature, this study, published in the prestigious journal *Science*, was the first description of a simple, reliable laboratory test to quantitate the growth-inhibiting potential of a drug against a human pathogen. Alexander's technique ultimately became the basis for the antibiotic susceptibility testing used today that guides physicians in choosing the most appropriate drug to treat patients with all bacterial infections, including meningitis.

After calculating the minimal effective concentration of streptomycin, Alexander proceeded to animal infection studies. She injected mice with *H. influenzae* and then treated them with the drug. To her deep satisfaction, relatively low doses of streptomycin successfully prevented infection in the mice. Further, these low dose results correlated well with her susceptibility assay results. Armed with that information, she proceeded to treat several of her *H. influenzae* meningitis patients with streptomycin. Their outcomes, particularly for patients treated early in their infections, were better than the treatment in use at that time, which was influenzal immune serum and a sulfa drug.[3]

Many antibiotics used today are manufactured in pharmaceutical chemistry laboratories by stitching together carbon, oxygen, hydrogen, nitrogen, and other elements into complex molecules that either kill or inhibit the growth of bacteria. For eons, however, antibiotics have been synthesized by bacteria and fungi that live deep in the dirt, where microorganisms of every ilk compete with each other for the local nutrients to survive. One of the microbes' offensive strategies is to launch chemical attacks on other microbes[4,5]—it's Mother Nature's gift to bacteria, a way to protect themselves from things that will harm them. Many of the attack substances deployed by the microbes have the ability to kill other bacteria; that is, they possess bactericidal activity and thus are antibiotics.

For nearly a century, physicians have serendipitously stumbled across these natural antibiotics and used them against bacteria that cause human infections. Penicillin, for example, was first discovered, although the scientists didn't realize the importance of their chance observations, by William Roberts in 1874 and John Tyndall in 1876 as a product of the mold *Penicillium glaucum* and then rediscovered by Alexander Fleming in 1929 as a product of *Penicillium notatum*.[6–9] Streptomycin, discovered by Schatz et al. in 1943, is produced by the bacteria *Streptomyces griseus*.[2] Erythromycin is produced by *Saccharopolyspora erythraea* (previously *Streptomyces erythraea*),[10] and tetracycline is produced by *Streptomyces aureofaciens*.[11]

Ancient bacteria not only produced antibiotics but also *ate* antibiotics. A number of bacterial species obtain nutrients for growth by ingesting antibiotic molecules present in their environment.[12] This phenomenon was first described by Y. Abd-el-Malek and colleagues as they studied decomposition of antibiotics. They percolated the antibiotic chloramphenicol through fresh garden soil from Cairo and discovered that the drug disappeared over several days. Among the many microbes in the Egyptian dirt, an unnamed *Streptomyces*-like bacterium was the only one associated with the disappearance of the chloramphenicol, and the *Streptomyces* used chloramphenicol as its sole source of the essential nutrients carbon and nitrogen.[13]

Further, microbes are able to *feel*, such that when they bump into a solid structure in their environment, their physiologic processes change, and they are able to stick to that structure through complex changes in their flagella and pili that result in new adherence organs, the holdfasts.[14]

Bacteria even *talk* to each other by a process called quorum sensing. They release diffusible signaling molecules that bind to receptors on other bacteria of the same species and trigger biochemical pathways with a number of biological functions—the higher the concentration of bacteria, the stronger the biologic action is.[15] This process was first discovered in *Aliivibrio fischeri* (formerly *Vibrio fischeri*), the bacteria that live in the nutrient-rich eye organ of Hawaiian bobtail squids.[16] When the bacteria reach a high enough density in the light organ of awake squids, the squid genes for producing bioluminescent (light-producing) molecules (luciferases) are turned on, and light shines from their ventral surfaces. The light thus emitted from the squids as they swim creates the appearance of sunlight filtered through the water and confuses their predators. When they are asleep, the squids eject most of the *Aliivibrio* bacteria, and no light is emitted.[17]

Through quorum-sensing signals, bacteria are able to alert each other when their population (i.e., the concentration of the signal molecules) is too dense or too sparse; thus, when necessary (e.g., under certain environmental conditions) they are able to make a change, such as initiate swarming behavior, activate virulence factors, or express host defense mechanisms. The bacteria that cause meningitis, *H. influenzae*, pneumococci, and meningococci, all possess quorum-sensing systems that regulate a large number of their bacterial functions. Further, bacteria often live in diverse communities with many other kinds of microbes and can eavesdrop on other bacteria by binding signaling molecules produced by their neighbors.[18-20] Some of those signaling molecules also function as antibacterial molecules.

Because Mother Nature provides microbes with the ability to make antibiotics, she also must give them antidotes to the antibiotics, correctives to prevent them from killing the organisms that produced them (i.e., a suicide), their close friends (i.e., a homicide), or relatives (i.e., a familicide).[21] Thus, nature bestowed on microbes the means to resist antibiotics. In his original paper describing penicillin, Fleming noted that his extract of the *P. notum* did not inhibit the growth of several bacteria, including *Bacillus influenzae* (as *H. influenzae* was called then) and *Bacillus coli* (now called *E. coli*).[8] Edward Abraham and Sir Ernst Boris Chain first discovered the mechanism for that inhibition when they observed that *B. coli* produced an enzyme, now known as penicillinase, that chemically degraded the penicillin.[22]

In addition to secreting enzymes that destroy specific antibiotics, microbes possess several other ways to resist the killing action of antibiotics. The permeability of their surface membranes may be altered so the antibiotics can't get inside. For example, gram-negative bacteria, such as *H. influenzae*, have both outer and inner membranes in their cell envelopes, which reduces access of some antibiotics to their targets in the interior of the bacterial cell.[23] Further, bacterial genes may occasionally acquire mutations that permit the microbes to survive and reproduce freely in new or changing environments. Such mutations may result in altered antibiotic target molecules (e.g., antibiotic receptors, enzyme substrates, etc.). For example, some strains of *H. influenzae* have acquired deformities in their surface proteins that bind penicillins such that penicillin-like antibiotics can't attach to the bacteria (Figure 9.1). The result is resistance to penicillin.[24]

Finally, bacteria may develop resistance to antibiotics by co-opting efflux pumps that were originally designed to flush toxic materials from the inside of the bacterial cell. Some of these pumps have evolved into siphons so that, once the antibiotics have entered the bacterial cells, the drugs drain back out before they can damage the bacteria (Figure 9.2).[25]

Resistance of human bacterial pathogens to antibiotics is strongly related to exposure of the microbes to antibiotics, but that doesn't occur exclusively in the setting of overuse, or even ordinary use, of antimicrobial drugs. Bacteria naturally resistant to antibiotics were found in the dirt from the Solomon Islands before antibiotics had ever been used in that locale; specifically, *E. coli* and an *Alcaligenes*-like organism produced factors that rendered them resistant to tetracycline and streptomycin.[26] In addition, DNA analysis of permafrost sediments from the

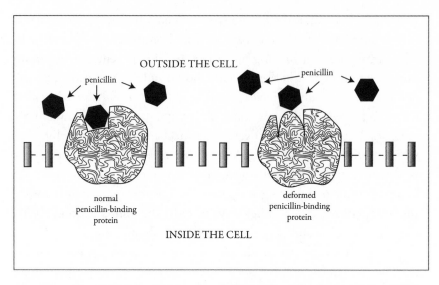

FIGURE 9.1 Antibiotic resistance by deformed antibiotic receptor. When the bacterial outer membrane protein that binds penicillin is mutated, penicillin is no longer able to nest in the protein's binding groove.

Drawing by the author.

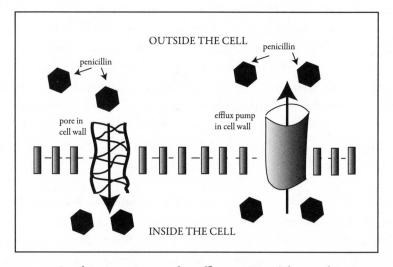

FIGURE 9.2 Antibiotic resistance by efflux pumps. The antibiotic enters the bacterial cell through a pore in the cell wall and is pumped back out via the efflux pump.

Drawing by the author.

Pleistocene Era at Bear Creek, near Dawson City, Yukon, revealed a number of genes that mediated antibiotic resistance (*vanX* [resistance to vancomycin], *bla* [resistance to penicillin], and *tetM* [resistance to tetracycline]).[27] The presence of these resistance genes, even before humans roamed Earth, represents successful adaptation on the part of bacteria to stressful conditions through which they acquired genetic mutations or new genetic elements that promoted their survival. Originally, these genes and their gene products very likely had a different purpose than resisting the action of antimicrobial agents and probably served a metabolic function of some sort.[28] Over the ages, ancient soil bacteria passed these genes to their offspring, as well as to neighboring bacteria through the process of horizontal gene transfer, until the genes were ultimately acquired by bacteria capable of causing infections in humans.

One of Hattie Alexander's patients was a previously healthy 2-year-old boy who had been "running about" the day before he became sick. When Alexander first examined him soon after his admission to the hospital, he was semicomatose, and his neck was stiff. His spinal fluid showed bacteria that looked like *H. influenzae* on Gram stain, and the sugar concentration was very low (6 mg%), suggesting he had severe meningitis. Alexander decided to treat him with streptomycin alone. She injected one dose into his cerebrospinal fluid and subsequent doses into his muscles. Within 24 hours, he was no longer disoriented, his fever had improved (from 104°F to 102°F), and his abnormal neurologic signs had not progressed. One day later, another spinal fluid specimen showed marked improvement as no bacteria were seen on stains, and the sugar content had returned to normal. His fever, however, had risen back to 104°F. On the third day, the spinal fluid culture obtained the day before was growing *H. influenzae*. His clinical status then rapidly deteriorated, and he developed right-side seizures and paralysis.[29] The antibiotic was no longer working. What had happened?

Many possibilities could explain why streptomycin failed to treat this child's *H. influenzae* meningitis:

1. The dose of the drug was too low.
2. Substances in the patient's body competed with the antibiotics and effectively neutralized their ability to kill the bacteria.

3. The streptomycin, given by muscle, failed to reach the meninges in high enough quantities to kill the bacteria that circulated in the fluid surrounding the brain.
4. The streptomycin had been stored inadequately and degraded in the bottle before the child received any of it.
5. The *H. influenzae* that infected the boy had become resistant to the bacterial killing effect of streptomycin.

Which possibility was it?

Alexander's young patient failed streptomycin treatment for his meningitis soon after scientists recognized the phenomenon of antibiotic resistance. Alexander and Grace Leidy, alarmed and puzzled by the drug failure, tested all the *H. influenzae* strains isolated from that child for their resistance to streptomycin. The bacteria obtained *before* he began streptomycin treatment were sensitive to the drug, but those obtained *after* initiation of treatment were highly resistant. In the minimal effective concentration assay, more than 1,000 units of streptomycin per milliliter of culture media, a massive dose, failed to kill the child's now streptomycin-resistant *H. influenzae*.[29] Clearly, the bacteria that caused his meningitis had become streptomycin resistant while he was being treated with that antibiotic.

Alexander considered two possible explanations for what had happened in this patient: (1) The *H. influenzae* that caused his infection had changed on exposure to the streptomycin, so the bacteria were now resistant, or (2) the *H. influenzae* that originally caused his infection consisted of two populations—a large number of bacteria that were susceptible to streptomycin, but a tiny fraction that were resistant—and on treatment with streptomycin, the resistant organisms managed to survive and then thrive while the sensitive organisms died.

To understand which option was correct, she cultured huge numbers of bacteria from 10 different streptomycin-susceptible *H. influenzae* strains, using agar that contained high levels of streptomycin. A few bacteria from each strain survived; between 0.07 and 1 in a billion bacteria were resistant. She concluded that after she had instituted streptomycin therapy for the boy's *H. influenzae* meningitis, the bacteria hadn't essentially changed, but rather the antibiotic treatment had

WHEN ANTIBIOTICS FAIL   177

killed all the susceptible bacteria in his spinal fluid, but left behind the very rare resistant ones. These resistant bacteria then multiplied and led to reemergence of the boy's meningitis symptoms. And, the *H. influenzae* multiplied quickly. Many bacteria replicate about every 20 minutes, so after an hour, 10 bacteria have become 80, and after 5 hours these have become 328,000.

Ultimately, things turned out well for Alexander's patient. When his fever escalated, she quickly recognized that the streptomycin treatment was no longer working, stopped it, and began treating the boy with the old therapy, immune serum and sulfadiazine. Within 3 days, he showed rapid improvement, and 4 weeks later, he was "walking around in his bed," could "move his arms normally," and appeared "to be normal mentally."[30]

Hattie Elizabeth Alexander (Figure 9.3) was born in 1901 in Baltimore, the second of eight children in a family of modest means.[31] In her early days, she loved athletics and found sports much more interesting than schoolwork.[32] Her grades were good enough, and her family's resources limited enough, that she qualified for a scholarship at Goucher College in Baltimore, where she was an "inconspicuous student."[31] After graduating, she worked as a bacteriologist for the Public Health Service for 3 years to earn money to continue her studies and then attended medical school at Johns Hopkins University. She excelled in her medical studies and received her MD degree in 1930. After completing her pediatric training at Columbia University in New York, she remained on the faculty there for the rest of her career.

Alexander's manner was formal and gruff, and she was viewed by the residents-in-training as inordinately critical of their clinical presentations during ward rounds. She often pelted them with questions like, "How do you know that?" "What is your evidence?" and "What makes you think so?"[33] Her constant drilling annoyed the residents and made her a frequent target of their Christmas party skits.[34] Her research work, however, was highly respected by her pediatric colleagues. In recognition of their esteem, they elected her as the first woman president of the American Pediatric Society, and the premier society for pediatric investigators awarded her the E. Mead Johnson award from the American Academy of Pediatrics.

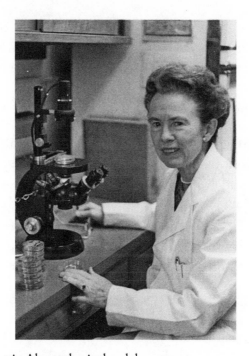

FIGURE 9.3 Hattie Alexander in her laboratory.

From the National Library of Medicine, National Institutes of Health. https://www.
nlm.nih.gov/changingthefaceofmedicine/physicians/biography_4.html.

It was relatively late in her professional life, at age 50, that she
began to study the molecular genetics of bacteria, which required her
to embrace new scientific concepts and to learn many new laboratory
techniques. After she identified the process of transformation (acqui-
sition of new DNA) in *H. influenzae* and defined the mechanism of
streptomycin resistance, she subsequently published papers on viral
RNA, bacterial DNA, and genetic heterogeneity in several additional
Haemophilus species.

Alexander never married, but lived for many years with Dr. Elizabeth
Ufford in Port Washington, Long Island, where she enjoyed growing
orchids in her greenhouse, listening to music on her "hi-fi,"[31] and
riding in her speedboat.[35] In her early 60s, she suffered a spontaneous
subarachnoid (brain) hemorrhage, which left her incapacitated for a
number of weeks, but she appeared to make a complete recovery. In her
mid-60s, she underwent a radical mastectomy for breast cancer, which,

unfortunately, recurred as metastases to her liver, from which she died in 1968 at age 67 years.[34]

Many scientists can claim one or possibly two very important discoveries in a lifetime. Alexander's notable discoveries number many more than that. Further, they emerged from her astute clinical observations and commitment to her patients as well as her deep understanding of microbiology and immunology and bacterial genetics. She pioneered the first medical therapy for *H. influenzae* meningitis but didn't stop when she learned that her immune serum improved the survival rate to nearly 60% because that wasn't good enough for her patients. She subsequently learned that treating patients with both immune sera and a sulfa drug further improved the patients' survival rate. Later, she found that streptomycin was even better, and when a patient failed streptomycin therapy, she figured out the mechanism for the resistance of *H. influenzae* to that antibiotic. Her work in DNA transformation in *H. influenzae* helped lay the groundwork for all future studies in bacterial molecular genetics.

One of the irritating characteristics of antibiotic resistance genes is that they don't stand still. Rather, they move. And, they move easily, from one bacterium to the next, much like the fleas that jump from your neighbor's poodle to your family setter. Antibiotic resistance genes, which have beguiling names such as New Delhi metallo-β-lactamase, extended-spectrum β-lactamase, carbapenem-hydrolyzing β-lactamases, or aminoglycoside acetyltransferases as well as *erm*(A), *mef*(A), *qnr* (S1), or *cat*(A), embed themselves into pieces of DNA such as plasmids (small circular pieces of DNA) or transposons (jumping genes) located outside bacterial chromosomes, and they travel. Further, as constituents of larger pieces of DNA, antibiotic resistance genes can be acquired, through the process of transformation, by certain bacteria, such as *H. influenzae*, pneumococci, and meningococci, just as spilled milk is soaked up by a sponge.

Because they travel with impunity, the antibiotic resistance genes are ubiquitous and dangerous. They shuffle among bacteria in gangs. Several unique resistance genes often live shoulder to shoulder on the plasmids that dwell in bacteria, thus yielding organisms that are simultaneously resistant to many different classes of antibiotics. These genes, aboard their resistant bacteria, trek from person to person in trains and planes and hospitals, are pushed from place to place by blowing winds and flowing water, and hitchhike to people on the fur and feathers of animals. Thus, resistance genes are carried around the world.[12] It's like evolution gone amok: Antibiotics are everywhere (in children attending daycare, in residents of nursing homes, in cattle feed, on fruit trees in commercial orchards, in fish farms), and they drive the survival of antibiotic-resistant bacteria. Microbes, after all, follow the Darwinian principle of survival of the fittest: In the presence of antibiotics, the most fit bacteria are those that most vigorously resist the action of the antibiotics. Unfortunately, successfully treating patients with infections caused by antibiotic-resistant bacteria is increasingly difficult, and this poses a major challenge to today's scientists and physicians and a serious hazard to their patients.

References

1. Spellberg B, Taylor-Blake B. On the Exoneration of Dr. William H. Stewart: Debunking an Urban Legend. *Infectious Diseases of Poverty.* 2013;2(1):3.

2. Schatz A, Bugie E, Waksman SA. Streptomycin, a Substance Exhibiting Antibiotic Activity Against Gram-Positive and Gram-Negative Bacteria. *Proceedings of the Society for Experimental Biology and Medicine.* 1944;55(1):66–69.

3. Alexander HE, Leidy G, Rake G, Donovick R. *Hemophilus influenzae* Meningitis Treated with Streptomycin. *Journal of the American Medical Association.* 1946;132(8):434–440.

4. Djordjevic SP, Stokes HW, Chowdhury PR. Mobile Elements, Zoonotic Pathogens and Commensal Bacteria: Conduits for the Delivery of Resistance Genes into Humans, Production Animals and Soil Microbiota. *Frontiers in Microbiology.* 2013;4:86.

5. Schmidt R, Cordovez V, de Boer W, Raaijmakers J, Garbeva P. Volatile Affairs in Microbial Interactions. *The ISME Journal.* 2015;9(11):2329–2335.

6. Roberts W. Studies on Biogenesis. *Philosophical Transactions of the Royal Society of London.* 1874;164:457–477.

7. Tyndall J. The Optical Deportment of the Atmosphere in Relation to the Phenomena of Putrefaction and Infection. *Philosophical Transactions of the Royal Society of London.* 1876;166:27–74.

8. Fleming A. On the Antibacterial Action of Cultures of a Penicillium, with Special Reference to Their Use in the Isolation of *B. influenzæ. British Journal of Experimental Pathology.* 1929;10(3):226–236.

9. Fleming A. Penicillin. Nobel Prize Lecture. 1945. https://www.nobelprize.
    org/prizes/medicine/1945/fleming/lecture/. Accessed January 2, 2017.
10. McGuire JM BR, Anderson RC, Boaz HE, Flynn EH, Powell HM, Smith
    JW. Ilotycin, a New Antibiotic. *Antibiotics and Chemotherapy (Northfield)*.
    1952;2(6):281–283
11. Darken MA, Berenson H, Shirk RJ, Sjolander NO. Production of
    Tetracycline by *Streptomyces aureofaciens* in Synthetic Media. *Applied
    Microbiology*. 1960;8(1):46–51.
12. Allen HK, Donato J, Wang HH, Cloud-Hansen KA, Davies J, Handelsman
    J. Call of the Wild: Antibiotic Resistance Genes in Natural Environments.
    Nature Reviews—Microbiology. 2010;8(4):251–259.
13. Abd-El-Malek Y, Monib M, Hazem A. Chloramphenicol, a Simultaneous
    Carbon and Nitrogen Source for a *Streptomyes* sp. from Egyptian Soil.
    Nature. 1961;189(4766):775–776.
14. Hughes KT, Berg HC. The Bacterium Has Landed. *Science*.
    2017;358(6362):446–447.
15. Ryan RP, Dow JM. Diffusible Signals and Interspecies Communication in
    Bacteria. *Microbiology*. 2008;154(7):1845–1858.
16. Nealson KH, Hastings JW. Bacterial Bioluminescence: Its Control and
    Ecological Significance. *Microbiological Reviews*. 1979;43(4):496–518.
17. Nyholm SV, McFall-Ngai M. The Winnowing: Establishing the Squid-
    Vibrio Symbiosis. *Nature Reviews—Microbiology*. 2004;2(8):632–642.
18. Swords W. Quorum Signaling and Sensing by Nontypeable *Haemophilus
    influenzae*. *Frontiers in Cellular and Infection Microbiology*. 2012;2:100.
    https://doi.org/10.3389/fcimb.2012.00100. Accessed January 10, 2017.
19. Cvitkovitch DG, Li Y-H, Ellen RP. Quorum Sensing and Biofilm
    Formation in Streptococcal Infections. *Journal of Clinical Investigation*.
    2003;112(11):1626–1632.
20. Winzer K, Sun Y-h, Green A, et al. Role of *Neisseria meningitidis* luxS in
    Cell-to-Cell Signaling and Bacteremic Infection. *Infection and Immunity*.
    2002;70(4):2245–2248.
21. Hopwood DA. How Do Antibiotic-Producing Bacteria Ensure Their Self-
    Resistance Before Antibiotic Biosynthesis Incapacitates Them? *Molecular
    Microbiology*. 2007;63(4):937–940.
22. Abraham EP, Chain E. An Enzyme from Bacteria Able to Destroy Penicillin.
    Reviews of Infectious Diseases. 1988;10(4):677–678.
23. Opal SM, Pop-Vicas A. Molecular Mechanisms of Antibiotic Resistance
    in Bacteria. In: Bennett JE, Dolin R, Blaser MJ, eds. *Mandell, Douglas,
    and Bennett's Principles and Practice of Infectious Diseases* (8th ed.).
    Philadelphia: Elsevier-Saunders; 2015:235–251.
24. Tristram S, Jacobs MR, Appelbaum PC. Antimicrobial Resistance in
    Haemophilus influenzae. *Clinical Microbiology Reviews*. 2007;20(2):368–389.
25. Barrett TC, Mok WWK, Brynildsen MP. Biased Inheritance Protects Older
    Bacteria from Harm. *Science*. 2017;356(6335):247–248.

26. Gardner P, Smith D, Beer H, Moellering R. Recovery of Resistance (R) Factors from a Drug-Free Community. *The Lancet.* 1969;294(7624):774–776.

27. D'Costa VM, King CE, Kalan L, et al. Antibiotic Resistance Is Ancient. *Nature.* 2011;477(7365):457–461.

28. Martinez JL, Fajardo A, Garmendia L, et al. A Global View of Antibiotic Resistance. *FEMS Microbiology Reviews.* 2009;33(1):44–65.

29. Alexander HE, Leidy G. Mode of Action of Streptomycin on Type b *H. influenzae. The Journal of Experimental Medicine.* 1947;85(4):329–338.

30. Alexander HE, Leidy G. Influence of Streptomycin on Type b *Haemophilus influenzae. Science.* 1946;104(2692):101–102.

31. Ligon BL. Hattie Alexander, MD: Pioneer Researcher. *Seminars in Pediatric Infectious Diseases.* 2000;11(2):155–158.

32. National Library of Medicine. Dr. Hattie Elizabeth Alexander. Changing the face of Medicine. 2003. https://www.nlm.nih.gov/changingthefaceofmedicine/physicians/biography_4.html. Accessed December 11, 2016.

33. Christy N. Hattie E. Alexander 1901–1968. *Physicians and Surgeons Journal.* 1997;17(2):1–2.

34. McIntosh R. Hattie Alexander. *Pediatrics.* 1968;42(3):544–544.

35. Columbia University Health Sciences Library Archives. Hattie Alexander Papers. 2005. http://library-archives.cumc.columbia.edu/finding-aid/hattie-alexander-papers-1939-1981. Accessed December 11, 2016.

10

Keeping DNA Out, Letting It In

FROM TIME TO TIME, people get infections with viruses (think colds and flu). So do dogs (think parvovirus and kennel cough), bees (deformed wing virus), and mosquitoes (baculoviruses). Microbes also get viral infections. The viruses that infect, and reproduce within, bacteria are known as bacteriophages (meaning bacteria eaters) and essentially are packets of DNA (or rarely RNA) on spider-like legs. Just as Mother Nature provides humans with ways to protect themselves from bacteria and viruses (i.e., antibodies, complement, white blood cells, etc.), she does the same for bacteria. Her antiviral gift to bacteria are genetic scissors that cut foreign DNA, such as the DNA in viruses that try to infect bacteria, into little pieces (Figure 10.1). Similar to cutting up a shoestring, cutting the strands of DNA from bacteriophages renders them unable to function properly.

A word about DNA: Deoxyribonucleic acids (DNAs), large molecules that carry genes on the chromosomes of living cells, are composed of threads of smaller molecules called nucleotides. Each nucleotide is composed of a sugar (deoxyribose), a phosphate, and one of four bases abbreviated by their first letters: A = adenine, T = thymidine, C = cytosine, G = guanine. The nucleotides are strung together like pearls on a cord, and the order of the bases in each chain determines the "genetic code" that instructs the cell's machinery to make the specific proteins important in cellular activities, such as physiologic processes, growth, and differentiation. Further, the nucleotide strands, like the stringers of a ladder,

Continual Raving: A History of Meningitis and the People Who Conquered It. Janet R Gilsdorf, Oxford University Press (2020). © Oxford University Press.
DOI: 10.1093/oso/9780190677312.001.0001

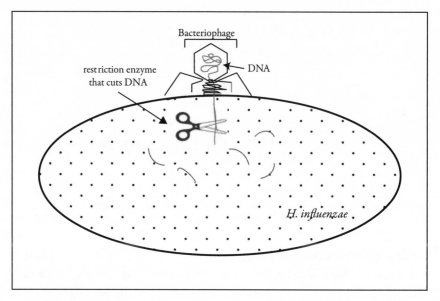

FIGURE 10.1 Restriction endonuclease of *H. influenzae* destroying DNA in a bacteriophage that has attacked the bacterium.
Drawing by the author.

are organized in pairs that serve as cross-links, like rungs, between the strands; A always binds to T and C always binds to G. For example,

5′ ATTGGCTCCATAGCTT 3′

| | | | | | | | | | | | | | | |

3′ TAACCGAGGTATCGAA 5′

By convention, the end of any nucleotide strand with a phosphate molecule is termed the 5′ end, while the end with a hydroxyl molecule, composed of hydrogen and oxygen, is termed the 3′ end. In the process of making proteins, the genetic code is read from the 5′ end to the 3′ end on each strand.

Haemophilus influenzae, and other bacteria that cause meningitis, have evolved genetic scissors to defang foreign DNA, such as that in viruses (bacteriophages) that attack them. The scissors are actually enzymes (biologically active proteins) produced by the bacteria. The hills, valleys, and folds (i.e., the physical conformation) of these enzymes match those of small stretches of DNA, allowing the enzymes and the nucleotides in the DNA to fit together like nesting teaspoons. For example, one of *H. influenzae*'s genetic scissors, called HindII (isolated from H. *influenzae* type d) wraps around the DNA's nucleotide sequence 5′-GT(T or C)(A or G)AC-3′ on one DNA strand and its corresponding sequence 3′-CA(A or G)(C or T)TG-5′ on the opposing DNA strand and causes each of the two DNA strands to break apart midway between those six nucleotides (Figure 10.2a). The specific nucleotide sequence on the DNA that the enzymes target is like an address that tells the HindII where to sit down and start cutting.

By breaking up the foreign DNA that invades the bacteria, the *H. influenzae* HindII enzymes limit, or *restrict,* the ability of DNA-containing bacteriophages to infect *H. influenzae* cells. Thus, these enzymatic scissors are also called restriction enzymes. The specific places on the strands of nucleotides where the enzymes cut the foreign DNA, which are unique to each enzyme, are called restriction sites.

Even though *H. influenzae* restriction enzymes cut DNA from viruses or other bacteria, they don't cut their own bacterial DNA. That's because Mother Nature, through evolution, has granted bacteria the means with which to prevent their self-destruction. *Haemophilus influenzae* decorate the restriction sites of their own DNA with chemicals called methyl groups (Figure 10.2b), and their genetic scissors can't cut through the methyl groups; it would be like trying to cut through a metal zipper.

This complex system of cutting up DNA and protecting against the cutting has formed the backbone of modern molecular genetics. DNA from any source can be cut into little pieces with restriction enzymes, and these pieces can be used for

molecular manipulation of bacteria and other living things;
determining the gene sequences of any DNA;
moving DNA from one bacterial cell to another;
repairing errors in DNA;
DNA analysis of criminal specimens;

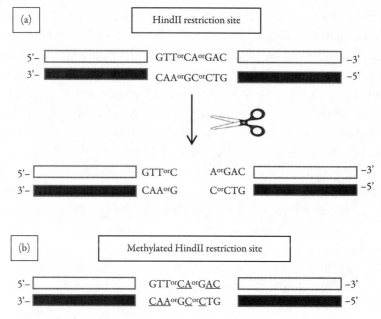

Underlined = methylated nucleotides

FIGURE 10.2   HindII endonuclease of *H. influenzae*. a. Cleavage of DNA at the restriction site. The space in the nucleotides below the scissors represents the site in the string of nucleotides where HindII endonuclease cuts. TorC, for example, reflects either the nucleotide T (thymidine) or C (cytidine) at this site. b. Methyl group modification protects cleavage of the restriction site.

Drawing by the author.

settling paternity suits by DNA analysis;
epidemiologic tracking of infectious diseases;
tracing the travels of ancient peoples;
and myriad other molecular applications.

In addition, these molecular tools have fostered the development of new vaccines against meningitis-causing bacteria.[1]

The restriction enzyme HindIII and related enzymes in *H. influenzae* were first identified by Dr. Hamilton Smith and his student Kent Wilcox (the paper describing this finding misspells the name as "Welcox"[2]) in 1970 in what Smith has called "a chance discovery,"[3] one of many that dotted his highly productive scientific career. When Smith first arrived at Johns Hopkins Medical School as a junior faculty member, he began to study genetic transformation—the transfer of genes from one microbe to another—in bacteria. In his experiments, he chose to use *H. influenzae* strain Rd, the unencapsulated Rough variant of a strain that formerly possessed a type d capsule. Smith had gotten the Rd strain from Dr. Roger Herriott, a biochemist across the street at the Johns Hopkins School of Hygiene and Public Health. Herriott had described the ideal growth medium to facilitate *H. influenzae* transformation, which ironically starves the bacteria.[4] Transformation occurs when bacteria are stressed, and starvation definitely taxes them. The *H. influenzae* that Smith used was the same Rd strain that Margaret Pittman had identified 40 years earlier as lacking a capsule.[5] Further, it was the same Rd strain that Hattie Alexander and Grace Leidy had used 20 years earlier to demonstrate that DNA from a strain with a type d capsule could transform an *H. influenzae* that had lost its capsule into one that had gained the type d capsule.[6]

To introduce young Wilcox to working with *H. influenzae*, Smith handed him a test tube containing DNA from bacteriophage P22, which Smith had studied prior to his arrival at Hopkins, and told the young graduate student to transform it into strain Rd. Wilcox gave it his best, but no matter what he did, strain Rd just wouldn't transform. The control *H. influenzae* DNA moved easily into strain Rd, but the phage DNA would not go. Smith assumed Wilcox had "bummed up the experiment in some way."[7] Rather than giving up on the student and the project, Smith reminded Wilcox of the article describing newly discovered restriction enzymes in *Escherichia coli* that he, Smith, had presented at the departmental journal club a week earlier.[8] He and Wilcox wondered if the failure of bacteriophage P22 DNA to transform into *H. influenzae* might be because the *H. influenzae* possessed a restriction enzyme that cut apart the phage DNA.

Restriction (i.e., the process by which bacteria cut apart, and don't take up, foreign DNA) had been described only in *E. coli*, and Smith thought such an explanation, from last week's journal club no less, of what they saw in *H. influenzae* would be too big a coincidence. Nevertheless, he and Wilcox devised a way to test the hypothesis. If the *H. influenzae* Rd possessed restriction enzymes, they reckoned, an extract of the bacteria would cut the phage P22 DNA into small fragments, which, in solution, would have lower viscosity (i.e., would be less gooey) than the larger, native DNA. They simply added a dollop of *H. influenzae* extract to bacteriophage P22 DNA, using the extract plus *H. influenzae*'s own DNA as a control, and drew the mixtures back and forth in the capillary tubes of their brand new viscometers to test their viscosity.

The two kinds of DNA, *H. influenzae* and P22, were the same size, so they should go through the little holes in the viscometer tubes identically. To their surprise, the mix with the *H. influenzae* DNA plus *H. influenzae* extract took much longer to go through the hole than the P22 DNA plus *H. influenzae* extract, indicating that the *H. influenzae* DNA was much larger than the P22 DNA. Something in the *H. influenzae* extract had changed the P22 DNA, but not its own DNA, and that something was the restriction enzyme HindIII. This discovery was a major breakthrough in understanding how, during the process of acquiring new genes, bacteria are selective about what they allow in and what they keep out.[9] Smith's discovery made all sorts of genetic engineering possible.

Hamilton Othanel Smith was born in 1931 in New York City, where his father was a doctoral student in education at Columbia University and his mother a teacher turned (not very successful) writer.[10] He and his older brother grew up in "an atmosphere of intense intellectualism," in which the boys received private French lessons, and young Ham studied the piano. Although he considered practicing to be a chore, he became a lifelong music lover after he stumbled across a recording of Arthur Rubenstein playing Beethoven's *Pathetique Sonata*. In spite of their interest in music, the Smith brothers used earnings from their paper route to stock the nascent chemistry-electronics laboratory in their basement. Ham described himself as having "kind of an inquiring mind" as a boy, for he "always wanted to know how things worked."[7(p. 1)]

After graduating from Johns Hopkins Medical School and completing his first year of medical internship at Barnes Hospital in St. Louis, Smith entered the US Navy. The United States had no universal draft at that time, but not enough physicians volunteered for military service, so a doctor draft had been established, and Ham's number was called. While serving as a general medical officer at Naval Base San Diego, California, he had Wednesday afternoons off and spent that time in the Endocrine Clinic, where he encountered patients with inherited disorders such as Turner and Kleinfelter syndromes. For the first time in years, he had time to relax and think and read, so he delved into the medical literature on genetic defects. He learned that people actually have 46 chromosomes rather than 48 as had been previously thought.[11] He taught himself to do squash preps, in which he placed a drop of a patient's blood on a slide, topped it with a glass coverslip, mashed it with his thumb, stained the now broken blood cells with orcein, and, examining them in a microscope, counted the chromosomes (Figure 10.3). Then, in 1957 and still in the navy, Ham read a genetics textbook by Theodosius Dobzhansky and learned about Watson and Crick and DNA.[12] He was hooked.

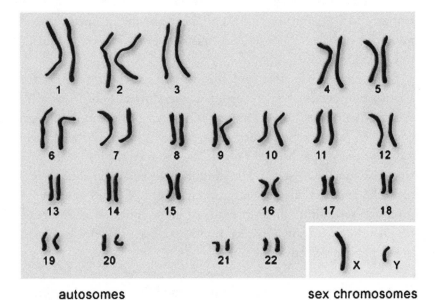

autosomes   **sex chromosomes**

FIGURE 10.3 Human chromosomes.

From US National Library of Medicine. How Many Chromosomes Do People Have? https://ghr.nlm.nih.gov/primer/basics/howmanychromosomes

During his subsequent medical residency at Ford Hospital in Detroit, Ham spent every spare hour in the library reading about bacteriophages and the chemical basis of heredity. He pored over copies of the *Journal of Molecular Biology*, including the one with François Jacob and Jacque Monet's article on the genetic control of enzyme and virus synthesis.[13] In his second year, one of his friends offhandedly mentioned that he was set to do a National Institutes of Health (NIH) research fellowship before entering medical practice.

Intrigued with the idea of learning to do research, Ham discussed it with his dad. Dr. Smith, the education professor, told his son of his recent visit to Ann Arbor, Michigan, to give a lecture. While waiting in the cafeteria line, he had stuck up a conversation with Dr. James Neel, the director of human genetics at the University of Michigan. The elder Smith suggested that Ham speak with Neel. Subsequently, Ham drove the 40 miles from Detroit to Ann Arbor to meet with Jim Neel, applied for an NIH fellowship award, was accepted, and began studying in Neel's genetics lab with a newly hired scientist, Dr. Mike Levine. From Levine, Smith learned to have fun working in a laboratory and experienced the joy of unearthing the mysteries of bacteriophage P22. Smith never considered returning to clinical medicine.

Smith has been described as a cheerful and soft-spoken man.[7] When I heard him present a guest lecture at the University of Michigan in the early 2000s, he was very upbeat as he described the molecular genetics of *H. influenzae* transformation. Actually, he exuded wild enthusiasm for everything he talked about and assumed the rest of the world would be equally as excited. His glorious smile and eager chuckle beckoned the audience into his magnificent world of genes and bacteria. Although serendipity directed many of his scientific successes, clearly his unending curiosity and keen mind have been significant cofactors in his highly productive career.

For his work on identifying the site on the DNA where the Hind restriction enzymes cleave, Smith, along with Werner Arber and Daniel Nathans, received the Nobel Prize in Medicine or Physiology in 1978 (Figure 10.4). In addition to Smith's work on the restriction enzymes, the award recognized his discovery that methylation of *H. influenzae*

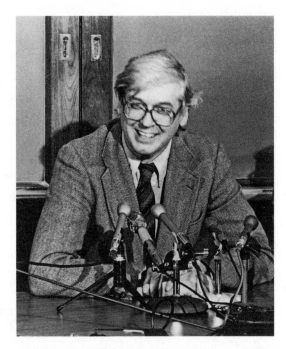

FIGURE 10.4 Hamilton Smith in a Nobel Prize press conference, 1978.
From US National Library of Medicine. The Daniel Nathans Papers. https://profiles.
nlm.nih.gov/ps/retrieve/Narrative/PD/p-nid/325/p-visuals/true
Photograph courtesy Susie Fitzhugh.

DNA, the addition of one carbon and three hydrogen atoms to the
DNA, protects it from digestion by its own restriction enzymes.[14,15]

Alike is boring—and unhealthy. *Different* promises resiliency and en-
sures survival. To be able to persist in the challenging environments
in which they find themselves, bacteria have to adapt to the frequent
changes in their surroundings. And, they adapt by diversification; that
is, among the large population of bacteria in a changing environment,
the few with unique, now favorable, genes (which direct the production
of favorable bacterial proteins) can survive. For the meningitis-causing
bacteria *H. influenzae*, pneumococci, and meningococci, diversification
allows them to continue to live in the many microniches of the human
pharynx. From there, they may squirm into the blood and circulate to
the brain, and the few that possess the "right stuff" for that environment are able to set up housekeeping in the cerebral meninges.

All bacteria have several strategies by which they diversify. Their DNA may be the victim of accidental mutations, in which a wrong nucleotide is mistakenly inserted into a gene, such as if an A is swapped for a G, when DNA divides. As a result, the mutated DNA makes an altered protein. While many such mutations are deleterious to bacteria, a few may be useful because they endow the bacteria with new, beneficial characteristics.

Bacteria may also diversify by acquiring new genes, the result of several different mechanisms: (1) They may become infected with viruses (i.e., bacteriophages) that insert new DNA into their cells; (2) pieces of DNA in transposons or plasmids that move from cell to cell may carry DNA from one bacterial cell to another; and, finally, (3) bacteria may undergo transformation, in which raw DNA floating in the environment burrows through the bacterial cell wall and into the cell's interior, where it attaches to the chromosome. Thus, transformation is essentially bacterial sex, the means by which individual bacteria acquire new DNA directly from other, usually related, bacteria. Unlike gene mutations or infection with a bacterial virus, gaining new, raw DNA by transformation doesn't occur by accident. Rather, it depends on highly evolved, highly coordinated molecular mechanisms.[16]

Hattie Alexander and Grace Leidy first demonstrated that an *H. influenzae* type b strain that lacked a capsule could be converted, or "transformed," into an *H. influenzae* with a different capsule type (a or c–f) by acquiring new DNA, and thus new genes, from a donor bacterial strain that possessed a non–type b capsule.[6] The cell envelopes of *H. influenzae*, however, are very impervious to things going in and things coming out. Like other gram-negative bacteria, their envelopes consist of outer and inner membranes composed of lipids (fats), sugars, and proteins. So, scientists asked, how exactly does the DNA get through the membranes and into the interior—that protected place where DNA normally resides on chromosomes—of bacterial cells?

The first glimpse into the mechanism of transformation in *H. influenzae* occurred when John Scocca and colleagues showed that only DNA from *H. influenzae* (or its cousin *Haemophilus parainfluenzae*) could be transformed into *H. influenzae* strain Rd. DNA from *E. coli* or from *Xenopus laevis*, which is a frog, would not go in.[17]

Shortly thereafter, Ham Smith and his colleagues hypothesized that *H. influenzae* DNA could be inserted into *H. influenzae* bacteria because of a specific interaction between the DNA and the bacterial cell. They digested *H. influenzae* DNA with a restriction enzyme from a different bacterium (*Bacillus amyloliquefaciens*) and observed that only a few of the resultant small DNA pieces were successfully taken up by *H. influenzae*.[18] Something was unique about those few transforming DNA pieces that made it in. What was it?

In subsequent experiments, Smith (Figure 10.5) and his students demonstrated that *H. influenzae* would only take up pieces of DNA that contained a string of 11 specific nucleotides.[19] Four years later, further experiments showed that it was actually nine nucleotides on the DNA that were the key to transformability: 5'-AAGTGCGGT-3'.[20] Such a sequence, which, along with its complimentary sequence on

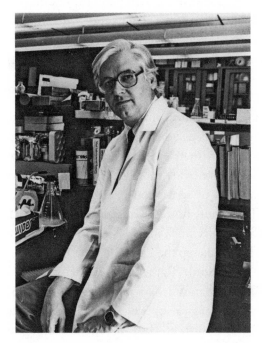

FIGURE 10.5 Hamilton Smith in the laboratory, 1978.

From US National Library of Medicine. The Daniel Nathans Papers. https://profiles. nlm.nih.gov/ps/retrieve/Narrative/PD/p-nid/325/p-visuals/true

Photograph courtesy Susie Fitzhugh.

the opposing nucleotide strand, must be present on a piece of DNA for successful transformation into *H. influenzae*. That magical sequence of nine base pairs is known as the DNA uptake signal sequence.

All three meningitis bacteria (meningococci, *H. influenzae*, and pneumococci) are able to soak up DNA from their environments; thus, they all exhibit substantial genetic diversity. Those whose cell walls stain gram negative (meningococci and *H. influenzae*) use DNA uptake signal sequences to take up the DNA, while pneumococci, which stain gram positive and thus possess a different kind of cell wall, use a unique, less well understood, mechanism.[21] Although these interesting and important scientific discoveries have little to do with the clinical management of meningitis, they reveal a lot about the basic biology of *H. influenzae* and other meningitis-causing bacteria. By using the molecular tools that permit bacteria to acquire new DNA from their environments, *H. influenzae* bacteria are able to refashion themselves. In this way, at least a few of the bacteria in the enormous population of bacteria that live in humans are able to cope with whatever challenging environment they happen to fall into, including their transit from the throat, where they normally live, to the blood and meninges, where they cause meningitis.

When Wilcox failed to transform bacteriophage P22 into *H. influenzae* bacteria, he and Smith decided the failure was explained by HindIII restriction enzymes in their *H. influenzae* extract that had cut up the P22 DNA. They proved this to be true and, for discovering HindIII and that entire class of restriction enzymes, Smith was awarded the Nobel Prize. Turns out, however, that although HindIII, indeed, digested the phage DNA in Wilcox's viscosity experiments, the reason *H. influenzae* didn't take up the P22 DNA had little to do with chewing up DNA (i.e., restriction).[7] Rather, as Smith later found out, that piece of phage P22 DNA that Wilcox tried to transform into *H. influenzae* did not possess the magical uptake signal sequence that would bind to the *H. influenzae* surface. Thus, it lacked the key to opening the transformation lock.

This new epiphany didn't diminish at all the scientific discoveries that earned Smith a well-deserved Nobel Prize, for the restriction enzymes he identified remained valid and important. Rather, it proved once again that even good people see only what they look for and, in doing so, may miss the rest of the beauty around them.

References

1. Serruto D, Bottomley MJ, Ram SJ, Giuliani MM, Rappuoli R. The New Multicomponent Vaccine Against Meningococcal Serogroup B, 4CMenB: Immunological, Functional and Structural Characterization of the Antigens. *Vaccine.* 2012;30(2):B87–B97.

2. Smith HO, Welcox KW. A Restriction Enzyme from *Hemophilus influenzae* I. Purification and General Properties. *Journal of Molecular Biology.* 1970;51(2):379–391.

3. Smith HO. Nucleotide Sequence Specificity of Restriction Endonucleases. Nobel Price Lecture. 1978. https://www.nobelprize.org/prizes/medicine/1978/smith/lecture/. Accessed February 15, 2017.

4. Herriott RM, Meyer EY, Vogt M, Modan M. Defined Medium for Growth of *Haemophilus influenzae. Journal of Bacteriology.* 1970;101(2):513–516.

5. Pittman M. Variation and Type Specificity in the Bacterial Species *Hemophilus influenzae. The Journal of Experimental Medicine.* 1931;53(4):471–492.

6. Alexander HE, Leidy G. Determination of Inherited Traits of *H. influenzae* by Desoxyribonucleic Acid Fractions Isolated from Type-Specific Cells. *The Journal of Experimental Medicine.* 1951;93(4):345–359.

7. Gitschier J. A Half-Century of Inspiration: An Interview with Hamilton Smith. *PLoS Genetics.* 2012;8(1):e1002466.

8. Meselson M, Yuan R. DNA Restriction Enzyme from *E. coli. Nature.* 1968;217(5134):1110–1114.

9. Kelly TJ, Smith HO. A Restriction Enzyme from *Hemophilus influenzae* II. Base Sequence of the Recognition Site. *Journal of Molecular Biology.* 1970;51(2):393–409.

10. Hamilton O. Smith—Facts. 1978. https://www.nobelprize.org/prizes/medicine/1978/smith/facts/. Accessed February 14, 2017.

11. Tjio JH, Levan A. The Chromosome Number of Man. *Hereditas.* 1956;42(1–2):1–6.

12. Dobzhansky T. *Evolution, Genetics and Man.* New York: Wiley; 1955.

13. Jacob F, Monod J. Genetic Regulatory Mechanisms in the Synthesis of Proteins. *Journal of Molecular Biology.* 1961;3(3):318–356.

14. Roy PH, Smith HO. DNA Methylases of *Hemophilus influenzae* Rd I. Purification and Properties. *Journal of Molecular Biology.* 1973;81(4):427–444.

15. Roy PH, Smith HO. DNA Methylases of *Hemophilus influenzae* Rd II. Partial Recognition Site Base Sequences. *Journal of Molecular Biology.* 1973;81(4):445–459.

16. Saunders NJ, Hood DW, Moxon ER. Bacterial Evolution: Bacteria Play Pass the Gene. *Current Biology.* 1999;9(5):R180–R183.

17. Scocca JJ, Poland RL, Zoon KC. Specificity in Deoxyribonucleic Acid Uptake by Transformable *Haemophilus influenzae. Journal of Bacteriology.* 1974;118(2):369–373.

18. Sisco KL, Smith HO. Sequence-specific DNA Uptake in *Haemophilus* Transformation. *Proceedings of the National Academy of Sciences of the United States of America.* 1979;76(2):972–976.

19. Danner DB, Deich RA, Sisco KL, Smith HO. An Eleven-Base-Pair Sequence Determines the Specificity of DNA Uptake in *Haemophilus* Transformation. *Gene.* 1980;11(3–4):311–318.

20. Fitzmaurice WP, Benjamin RC, Huang PC, Scocca JJ. Characterization of Recognition Sites on Bacteriophage HP1c1 DNA Which Interact with the DNA Uptake System of *Haemophilus influenzae* Rd. *Gene.* 1984;31(1–3):187–196.

21. Johnsborg O, Eldholm V, Håvarstein LS. Natural Genetic Transformation: Prevalence, Mechanisms and Function. *Research in Microbiology.* 2007;158(10):767–778.

11

Hitch a Sugar to a Protein

HOW CAN PARENTS PROTECT their children from meningitis? Unfortunately, simple solutions such as hand sanitizer, antiseptic soaps, mouthwash, or probiotics won't do it. While a well-balanced diet, exercise, creative play, and intellectual stimulation are important for good health in general, they don't prevent infections of the meninges. Meningitis in children is a rare chance event and mostly a matter of very bad luck. It occurs serendipitously after normal bacteria that live peacefully in a child's throat wrangle their way into the blood by largely unknown means and then flow with circulating blood, like leaves in a river, to the brain, where the bacteria cling to the meningeal tissues and cause meningitis. There is only one way to prevent meningitis. It is relatively easy and inexpensive, is definitely highly effective, and offers a strong antidote against the bad luck of meningitis. It's vaccination. While vaccines don't prevent all cases of meningitis in children, if used appropriately, they prevent nearly all.

How do vaccines work? They are essentially a twist on Trojan horses. The original Trojan horse, with Greek warriors concealed in its wooden belly, was viewed by the Trojans as a gift, foreign but benign. In truth, it wasn't benign at all. The invisible threat hidden inside the horse—soldiers ready to attack—fooled the Trojans into complacency and inaction. Vaccines, on the other hand, indeed, *are* benign, and are designed to fool our immune systems into thinking they've been attacked by a dangerous microbe and need to take action against that microbial threat. Vaccines,

Continual Raving: A History of Meningitis and the People Who Conquered It. Janet R Gilsdorf, Oxford University Press (2020). © Oxford University Press.
DOI: 10.1093/oso/9780190677312.001.0001

like microbes, contain immunogenic substances, or antigens, which our bodies recognize as foreign and then deploy powerful, protective immune factors, including antibodies, to counter the presumed assault.

The *ideal* vaccine, one that prevents infectious diseases such as meningitis, is composed of antigens that (1) stimulate a vigorous antibody response; (2) are exposed on the surface of the microbe so antibodies can bind to them; (3) are present in all disease-causing strains of the microbe; and (4) are immunologically identical on all strains. In addition, the ideal antigens must stimulate antibodies that kill, or neutralize, the microbe, and the resultant killing/neutralizing power of the antibodies must endure for the lifetime of the vaccine recipient. Finally, the ideal vaccine must be stable at room temperature, free of adverse reactions, and cheap and must require only one dose for lifelong immunity. As in all worldly domains, achieving the ideal is difficult. None of the current vaccines to prevent any disease meets all these criteria.

Bacterial (or viral) antigens that are used as vaccines can be almost any part of the microbe, from whole, intact bacteria or viruses to purified molecules that, in nature, are located on the microbe's surface; such antigens include proteins in bacterial cell envelopes or viral shells or the sugars that comprise bacterial capsules.[1] Sometimes the antigens are constituents of living microbial cells, sometimes of dead cells, sometimes of parts of cells. For living bacteria or viruses to be used as vaccines, they must be attenuated, or altered by heating or chemical treatments or genetic manipulation, to render them avirulent (unable to cause disease) and thus safe.

When Edward Jenner pioneered the use of cowpox scabs as a vaccine against smallpox, he relied on the relatively low virulence of the cowpox virus, as compared to the highly virulent smallpox virus, to ensure vaccine safety. Thus, he took advantage of an experiment of nature: the differential virulence of those two similar viruses.

It was the chemist and microbiologist Louis Pasteur, however, who first deliberately attenuated live viruses by physical means for use as vaccines. To prepare his vaccine against rabies, Pasteur obtained live rabies viruses from the saliva of rabid dogs, which wasn't easy (Figure 11.1). From Vallery-Radot's description of Pasteur's tenacity at obtaining saliva from a rabid dog, Percy and Mrs. Frankland reported,

They started, taking six rabbits with them in a basket. The rabid beast was in this case a huge bull-dog, foaming at the mouth and howling in his cage. All attempts to induce the animal to bite, and so infect one of the rabbits, failed; "but we *must*," said Pasteur, "inoculate the rabbits with this saliva." Accordingly, a noose was made and thrown, the dog secured and dragged to the edge of the cage, and his jaws tied together. Choking with rage, the eyes bloodshot, and the body

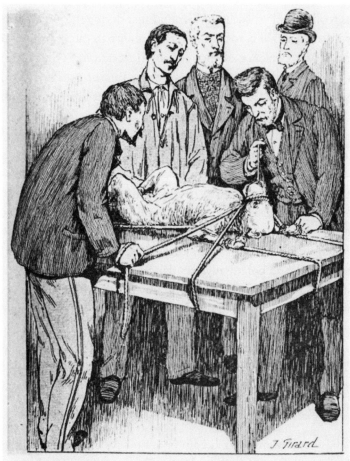

M. Pasteur aspirait, à l'aide d'un tube effilé, quelques gouttes de bave.

FIGURE 11.1 Pasteur obtaining saliva from a rabid dog.
From Lemoyne P. *Pasteur*. Abbeville, France: Paillart; 1900.
Drawing by J. Gerard.

convulsed by a violent spasm, the animal was stretched on a table, and kept motionless whilst Pasteur, leaning over this foaming head, sucked up into a narrow glass tube some drops of the saliva.[2(p. 167)]

Pasteur figured that since the rabies viruses survived and caused disease in the brains of infected humans and animals, they must reproduce readily in the tissues of the nervous system. Thus, to increase the number of infectious viruses for use in the vaccine, he injected the rabies virus–containing dog saliva into the spinal cords of rabbits and let the viruses replicate. He subsequently found that drying the viruses from the rabies-infected spinal cords reduced their ability to cause disease (i.e., he attenuated the virulence of the virus by desiccation).[2] After testing his vaccination procedure in rabbits and dogs, Pasteur was ready to inject pieces of rabies-infected rabbit spinal cords into the first human subject.[3]

On July 4, 1885, nine-year-old Joseph Meister was bitten at least 14 times by a rabid dog near his home in Alsace. His mother, terrified her son would die, begged her doctor to help him. The doctor told her about Pasteur, who was researching a treatment for rabies. Two days after the dog bite, Mme. Meister and young Joseph traveled to Paris in search of a cure. As reported by Rene Vallery-Radot, a writer and Pasteur's son-in-law, Pasteur was hesitant to subject healthy-appearing Joseph to the inadequately tested, and potentially very dangerous, rabies virus in his vaccine preparation. Two physician friends of Pasteur, however, recognized the risk of both the number and depth of the child's bite wounds and counseled Pasteur that Joseph, beyond a doubt, would eventually succumb to rabies. Reluctantly, Pasteur agreed to inoculate the boy with his new vaccine. The plan was to start the injections with very small doses of avirulent rabies viruses and gradually increase the potency of the vaccine.[4]

In the words of Pasteur's son-in-law,

As the inoculations were becoming more virulent, Pasteur became a prey to anxiety; "My dear children," wrote Mme. Pasteur, "your father has had another bad night; he is dreading the last inoculations on the child." ... Pasteur was going through a succession of hopes, fears, anguish, and an ardent yearning to snatch little Meister from death; he could no longer work. At night, feverish visions came to

him of this child whom he had seen playing in the garden, suffo-
cating in the mad struggles of hydrophobia, like the dying child he
has seen at the Hôpital Trousseau in 1880.[4(p. 416)]

The vaccination procedure proceeded without difficulty (Figure 11.2).
After receiving 13 injections of the vaccine, Joseph left Paris to return to
his home with instructions to report back to Pasteur daily. Sometimes

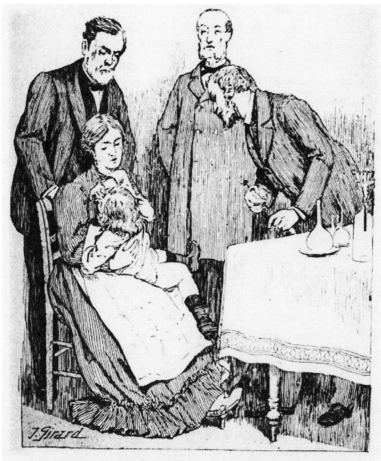

Inoculation du vaccin antirabique sur le jeune Joseph Meister.

FIGURE 11.2 Joseph Meister receiving the rabies vaccine.
From Lemoyne P. *Pasteur*. Abbeville, France: Paillart; 1900.
Drawing by J. Gerard.

5 or 6 days passed with no word from the Meisters, which tormented Pasteur. Was Joseph all right? Had he developed rabies from the vaccine? Or from the dog bites? Finally, a month after returning to Alsace, the boy wrote that he was well.

Although Pasteur obviously hadn't included a control in the experiment (i.e., a child who received a mock vaccine after being bitten by a rabid dog), he declared the rabies vaccine a success.

Employing living viruses from cowpox scabs or from rabies-infected rabbit spinal cords as vaccine antigens, such as Jenner and Pasteur did to prevent smallpox and rabies, respectively, was tedious and potentially dangerous and offered no consistency between vaccine batches. Thus, scientists began exploring methods that were easier and safer and yet provided reliable antigenic material that would induce strong immune responses in the vaccine recipients. If viruses could be propagated in the laboratory, many of those problems would be solved.

This was finally accomplished when John Enders and colleagues, in a major scientific breakthrough, demonstrated that polioviruses could reproduce in the laboratory when incubated in living cells obtained from the skin, muscle, and connective tissues of human embryos. Further, Enders and others successfully attenuated the virulence of the laboratory-grown viruses by serially cultivating them, over and over, in living cells.[5] During this process of "passing," the viruses became avirulent by either loss or modification of their virulence genes.[6] Thus, live viruses, such as measles, mumps, rubella, and varicella, which causes chickenpox, were subsequently attenuated for use as vaccines.[7–10]

Live virus vaccines pose the potential, albeit rare, danger of the vaccine viruses causing infection in the vaccine recipients. Thus, vaccines consisting of killed viruses have been studied extensively. Many didn't work very well. The killed measles vaccine, which did not stimulate good immune responses, was associated with atypical measles symptoms when the vaccine recipients encountered wild measles and was, thus, in 1967 withdrawn from the market.[11] Examples of killed virus antigens that offer good protection are the vaccines against Japanese encephalitis and hepatitis A.[12,13]

Both live and killed polioviruses are important in the conquest of poliomyelitis. The initial polio vaccine, licensed in the United States in

1955, utilized the killed poliovirus developed by Jonas Salk. The vaccine contained three types of polio virus, types 1, 2, and 3, which had been grown in monkey kidney cells and inactivated with formaldehyde.[14] This injectable vaccine was highly successful, as it reduced polio from 13.9 to 0.8 cases/100,000 people annually in the United States.[15]

It was the Salk vaccine I received as a Polio Pioneer in Cass County, North Dakota. My parents enrolled me in the massive polio vaccine trial of 1954, led by Dr. Tommy Francis of the University of Michigan School of Public Health.[16] I vividly remember standing in line with other third graders in the basement of Horace Mann Elementary School and breathing the ominous smell of rubbing alcohol. I was terrified of the impending "shot," yet was somehow aware that I was part of something really important. Before the polio vaccine, my mother wouldn't let me go to the swimming pool or to a parade during the summer for fear I'd contract the dreaded polio. That had happened to the neighbor boy who lived three blocks from my house. I used to stand on the sidewalk beside his open window, watch the curtains flapping in the breeze, and listen to the whoosh-whoosh of his iron lung.[17] After the vaccine came to our town, Mother's worries evaporated.

Subsequently, an attenuated virus, contained in the live virus polio vaccine developed by Albert Sabin, was found to be superior to the killed virus as a vaccine because the live virus was able to spread to, and immunize, unvaccinated contacts of the vaccinees.[18] The result of this research was the oral polio vaccine, originally delivered as pink liquid soaked into white sugar cubes, and widely used in the United States from 1963 to the 1990s.

By the 1990s, polio from wild-type viruses was rare in the United States. More common, however, was polio caused by live vaccine viruses that had become again virulent. Thus, in industrialized countries the Sabin live virus oral vaccine has been abandoned, and the Salk killed virus injected vaccine is now used exclusively.

In addition to whole viruses, vaccine antigens may also consist of individual proteins isolated from viruses. The original vaccine against hepatitis B consisted of a protein on the surface of the virus; the protein was named the Australia antigen because it was first discovered in the blood of an Australian Aborigine with chronic hepatitis B.[19,20] This protein, now known as hepatitis B surface antigen (HBsAg), was shed from the virus into the patient's blood. To produce the original vaccine, Maurice Hilleman and colleagues isolated Australia antigens from the plasma of people chronically infected with hepatitis B.[21] That plasma-derived vaccine, which ran the risk of containing as yet unknown viruses, was replaced by subsequent hepatitis B vaccines, which were the first to be prepared by recombinant DNA technology. To make the recombinant vaccine, Pablo Valenzuela and colleagues inserted a plasmid (a ring of DNA) carrying the gene that codes for the HBsAg protein into baker's yeast (*Saccharomyces cerevisiae*), and the genetically modified yeast cells began churning out HBsAg protein.[22] The protein was then isolated from the yeast, purified, and absorbed to an aluminum-containing adjuvant to improve the potency of the vaccine's immune response.[23]

More recently, Drs. Douglas Lowy, John Schiller, and colleagues developed a vaccine against human papilloma virus (HPV) composed of virus-like particles that contain the external viral capsid protein (named L1) without the internal DNA of the virus.[24] In recognition of this unique approach to preventing cancers caused by HPV, Lowy and Schiller received a 2017 Lasker Award.[25]

Antigens from bacteria have also been used as vaccines to protect against bacterial infections. Emil Von Behring and Shibasaburo Kitasato first taught the world that bacterial toxins, which are proteins, are useful vaccine antigens. They immunized rabbits against the toxins of the bacteria that cause tetanus and demonstrated that the resultant immune sera neutralized the noxious effects of tetanus toxin in mice and prevented death in mice challenged with tetanus-causing bacteria.[26] In the 1920s, Alexander Thomas Glenny and Barbara Hopkins as well as Pierre Descombey detoxified diphtheria and tetanus toxins, respectively, with formaldehyde, turning them into immunogenic, toxin-like proteins called toxoids, which were much safer as vaccines than the raw toxins.[27,28] The diphtheria and tetanus toxoid vaccines are still used today and are included in the routine vaccine series for infants and children.

The first vaccine against pertussis (whooping cough) utilized whole *Bordetella pertussis* bacteria inactivated with formaldehyde.[29] The diphtheria and tetanus toxoids and the whole-cell pertussis vaccines were combined into the DPT vaccine in 1948, which was used in the United States into the mid-1990s.

That old pertussis vaccine consisted essentially of –washed and chemically killed bacterial cells and beleaguered its young recipients with frequent, unpleasant side effects. Ultimately, new vaccines, the so-called acellular pertussis vaccines, consisting of either three or five purified *B. pertussis* proteins depending on the vaccine preparation, were licensed in the United States.[30] The acellular pertussis antigens have been combined with diphtheria and tetanus toxoids to become the DTaP vaccines—the "a" is for acellular. While causing fewer and milder adverse reactions compared to the whole-cell vaccine, the acellular pertussis vaccines, unfortunately, produce shorter-lived protection. Other components of the washed bacteria used in the old whole-cell vaccine, especially the endotoxins that likely contributed to the frequent side effects, probably acted as adjuvants to prolong the immune response. Consequently, additional booster doses of acellular pertussis vaccines are now recommended for pregnant women to prevent pertussis in their newborn babies and for adolescents.[31]

Initial attempts to prevent pneumococcal infections used a vaccine developed in the early 1900s composed of heat-killed *Streptococcus pneumoniae* bacteria. Doses of extremely high levels of bacteria (i.e., 1,000 and 2,500 million pneumococci) worked best to prevent pneumonia and death among the Rand coal miners of the South African Transvaal province.[32,33] Yet, the magnitude of the protection wasn't very good, likely because antibodies against the immunizing strain—they apparently used only one strain, whose capsule type wasn't known—wouldn't protect against infection by the many strains with different capsule types.[32] Thus, the original pneumococcal vaccines, which consisted of killed, whole bacteria, didn't work well and were not widely used.

The capsules that surround the meningitis bacteria (pneumococci, *H. influenzae*, and meningococci) are webs of long sugar molecules that protect the bacteria from being eaten and killed by white blood cells. William Tilletts and Thomas Francis first injected the polysaccharide capsules from pneumococci into humans as a vaccine, and blood drawn from the volunteers showed evidence of immune responses.[34]

Subsequently, several groups of scientists purified the capsules from pneumococci and tested them as vaccines. Indeed, the polysaccharide (sugar) antigens in the capsules induced high levels of antibodies in the adults tested and protected vaccine recipients against pneumococcal infection.[35–38] The early pneumococcal capsule vaccines were abandoned in the 1940s, however, because the emerging antibiotic drugs treated pneumococcal infections so successfully.

Pneumococcal capsule vaccines reemerged in the 1970s in the form of multivalent vaccines containing first 14 and subsequently 23 different capsule types.[39] Such vaccines don't, however, protect against all possible capsule types because, through the years, scientists have discovered more and more new, immunologically distinct pneumococcal capsule types. Presently, at least 97 unique serotypes have been described.[40]

From these studies with pneumococci, the notion of using polysaccharide capsule antigens as vaccines was extended to meningococci.[41,42] Ultimately, quadrivalent vaccines containing the capsules of serogroup A (which causes epidemic infections in sub-Saharan Africa), serogroup Y, and serogroup W as well as serogroup C (which cause many of the meningococcal infections in industrialized nations) were developed and licensed in 1981 in the United States.[43] While strains possessing the serogroup B capsule most commonly cause meningococcal infection in the United States, that specific polysaccharide capsule has not been pursued as a vaccine antigen because it consists of a form of sialic acid that is found on many human cells.[44] The human immune system would recognize that particular sialic acid–containing antigen as "self" rather than "foreign" and wouldn't generate an immune response. And, more worrisome, if it did, the antibodies might attack the sialic acid molecules on many human cells and organs, resulting in autoimmune disease.

Stephen Zaminoff and colleagues described the chemical nature (i.e., repeating sugar molecules) of the *H. influenzae* type b (Hib) capsule in 1953,[45] but it wasn't until the early 1970s that Dr. Rachel Schneerson and Dr. Porter Anderson injected the Hib capsule into adults and demonstrated its ability to generate antibodies.[46,47] With this information in hand, vaccines composed of the purified Hib capsule were developed and first licensed in the United States in 1985.[48] Anderson's vaccine contained the capsule purified from *H. influenzae* strain Eagan, originally obtained from a child, likely with the last name of Eagan, suffering from meningitis in Boston.[47] Schneerson's vaccine contained a pool of type b capsules isolated from strains from several patients; the largest component of the pool was the exceptionally abundant capsule from strain Rab (for Rabinowitz, a child with *H. influenzae* meningitis), which had originally been studied by Hattie Alexander and Grace Leidy.[49] As an aside, the capsules of the other *H. influenzae* types, a and c–f, haven't yet been studied widely as vaccine antigens, primarily because invasive infections with these forms of *H. influenzae* are very uncommon.

The Hib capsule is complex, and its chemical name, polyribophosphate (also known as polyribose phosphate, polyribosyl phosphate, or PRP) reflects its repeating units of the sugar ribose decorated with phosphate molecules (Figure 11.3). Its molecular weight is 362.224 g/mol. The

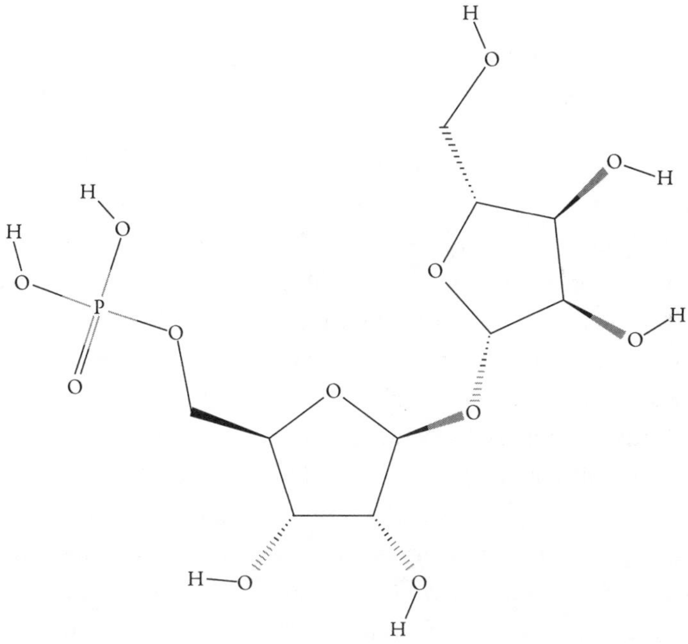

FIGURE 11.3 Chemical structure of *H. influenzae* type b capsule, polyribophosphate.

From National Center for Biotechnology Information. Compound Summary: Polyribophosphate. PubChem Compound Database CID = 123744. https://pubchem. ncbi.nlm.nih.gov/summary/summary.cgi?cid=123744.

chemical formula for the compound is $C_{10}H_{19}O_{12}P$.[50] The capsules of all type b strains are chemically and immunologically identical.

The problem with the *H. influenzae* PRP vaccine was that infants and young children can't make high levels of long-lasting antibodies against polysaccharide antigens, as was suggested almost 40 years earlier by Fothergill and Wright in their famous graph of age and immunity.[51] The reason for this failure rests in the complexity of the human immune system. In babies, immature plasma cells—the B-lymphocyte cells of the spleen and lymph nodes that produce antibodies—receive and process molecular signals from the regulatory T lymphocytes differently from mature plasma cells of older children and adults. As a result, the low levels of antipolysaccharide antibodies produced by young children are short-lived and aren't readily boosted by subsequent exposure to the polysaccharide antigen. Thus, infants and young children, who have the highest incidence of Hib meningitis, couldn't make protective antibodies against the capsular antigen contained in the first Hib vaccines.[52–54] The world needed a better vaccine for the babies.

In the quest to develop optimal vaccines to prevent Hib meningitis, two research teams led the way. They worked in parallel and, while they respectfully credited each other's work,[55] in many ways they were fierce competitors for the holy grail—an Hib vaccine that would protect babies. At the National Institutes of Health (NIH) in Bethesda, Maryland, one group, cramped in extremely crowded laboratories that teemed with postdoctoral trainees from around the world, was led by Dr. John B. Robbins, a pediatrician who was passionate about producing vaccines against all sorts of bacterial capsules, and Rachel Schneerson, who also trained as a pediatrician but worked as an immunochemist. The other group, originally at Harvard University and later at the University of Rochester, was led by Dr. David Smith, a pediatrician motivated to prevent *H. influenzae* infections after taking care of too many children with meningitis at Boston Children's Hospital, and Porter Anderson, a microbiologist turned chemist.

John Bennett Robbins (Figure 11.4), originally from Brooklyn, was a capsule antigen generalist, interested in the capsules of many different

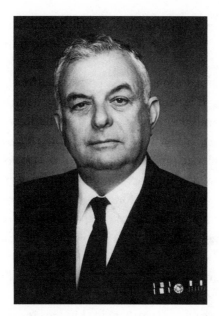

FIGURE 11.4 John B. Robbins, MD.
Courtesy of the Albert and Mary Lasker Foundation.

bacteria. After graduating from medical school at New York University and completing his residency in pediatrics in Boston, he joined the faculty of the University of Florida and, later, Albert Einstein University. In 1970, he moved to the NIH, where he spent the later part of his scientific career as director of the Laboratory of Developmental and Molecular Immunity, developing vaccines against capsules of many bacteria, including one against Hib. Besides his expertise in science, Robbins is reported to possess an encyclopedic knowledge of baseball, particularly all things related to the Brooklyn Dodgers, and he is an ardent connoisseur of Oriental rugs.[56]

Robbins is noted for his generosity, as evidenced by his readiness to supply valuable reagents to anyone who asked. In fact, I still have, in my laboratory freezer, a vial of *H. influenzae* anti-PRP serum from the infamous Burro 132 that he sent to me years ago. That burro had been immunized with *H. influenzae* strain Rab, and investigators, myself included, used the resultant antibodies to identify type b strains and to test bacteria for PRP antibody-mediated killing. Robbins reportedly distributed 173 liters of serum "from this remarkable beast."[56]

I recall Robbins as a loquacious fellow, one who still carries his Brooklyn accent and whose mind cannot be caged. I first met him at an infectious diseases meeting in St. Louis in about 1980—he was a luminary in our field and I, a pediatric infectious diseases fellow-in-training. When I boarded the shuttle bus from the hotel to the convention center, the only empty seat was beside Robbins. He chatted about the meeting, and the conversation drifted to a talk he was scheduled to give later in the day. He confessed to troublesome symptoms he always developed before speaking, characterized by raging gastrointestinal upset. I, of course, suffered anxiety before giving talks because I was relatively new at it, but I couldn't imagine an experienced, very famous, professional speaker like him with such a problem. I also couldn't understand why he told *me* about it. In the end, his presentation was excellent with no external evidence of the internal upset that had likely dogged him before he ascended the stage.

Robbins' decades-long partner in his vaccine work was Rachel Schneerson (Figure 11.5), who was born in Warsaw, Poland, and educated in Israel.[57] From 1968 until their retirement in 2012, she and

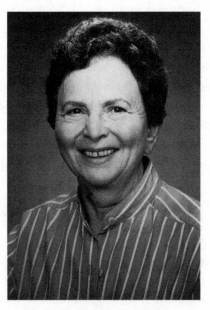

FIGURE 11.5 Rachel Schneerson, MD.
Courtesy of the Albert and Mary Lasker Foundation.

Robbins worked together on the development of many vaccines, such as those against cholera, *Salmonella*, pneumococci, meningococci, *E. coli*, *Staphylococcus aureus*, group B streptococci, and *Shigella*. During my visit to their laboratory at the NIH, I found Schneerson to be a very quiet, intense, private woman with a pleasant, ready smile. She always let Robbins do the talking.

In contrast to Robbins, the vaccine generalist, David Hamilton Smith, MD, who was born in Canton, Ohio, was a vaccine superspecialist, focused solely on finding a way to prevent *H. influenzae* meningitis in young children. His inspiration began while he was a house officer at Boston Children's Hospital. Reportedly, while making ward rounds with the pediatrics team, Dr. Charles Janeway, the legendary head of pediatric infectious diseases at the time, stopped at the bedside of a child with Hib meningitis and said to the trainees gathered around him, "One of you should try to find a vaccine to prevent this terrible disease."[58] David Smith (Figure 11.6) accepted the challenge. After a stint in the army, he completed a postdoctoral fellowship in molecular genetics and bacteriology at Boston Children's Hospital, where he

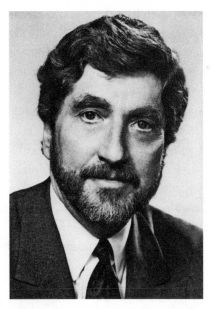

FIGURE 11.6 David Smith, MD.
Courtesy of the Albert and Mary Lasker Foundation.

ultimately became chief of pediatric infectious diseases. In 1968, he and Porter Anderson began the search for a vaccine against Hib.

In 1976, Smith moved to the University of Rochester as chair of the Department of Pediatrics, where he and Anderson continued their vaccine investigations. "Trying to come up with a vaccine for a bacterial disease in the late '60s was pretty lonely work," Smith is reported to have said.[59] The NIH and the drug companies were only interested in funding research into new antibiotics. By 1980, Smith and Anderson had developed a prototype *H. influenzae* vaccine but were unable to convince a pharmaceutical company to manufacture it. Infuriated, Smith resigned his position at the University of Rochester and started his own company, Praxis Biologics, originally housed in "a closet" in Rochester with only a few employees. As described by his wife, "He quit his job and mortgaged the house and founded the company."[59] He knew little about running a company and learned to write a business plan from books he checked out of the local library.[60] The vaccine ultimately came to market and became a huge clinical, and financial, success.

From observing him at scientific meetings, I remember David as a somewhat aloof, serious, highly focused scientist with tired eyes who commanded the room merely by his presence. In later years, while living on Martha's Vineyard, he became mindful of nature's fragility and made major contributions to the Polly Hill Arboretum and to the Nature Conservancy.[58] Sadly, David died in 1999 of malignant melanoma at the relatively young age of 67 years.

Porter Warren Anderson, Jr. (Figure 11.7), David Smith's sidekick in the discovery of the *H. influenzae* vaccine, was raised in Alabama and has been described as a cross between a polymath and a Renaissance man. While majoring in chemistry at Emory University he also studied history, Shakespeare, and music; played on the tennis team; and became acutely disturbed by the injustices of racism and anti-Semitism. A principled man, he resigned from his fraternity because he "came to think of it as a waste of time and money, and an influence for bad conduct."[61] After receiving his PhD in microbiology from Harvard, he taught for 2 years at the predominantly black Stillman College in Tuscaloosa, Alabama, but quit because he "disliked the Sisyphean quality of teaching, and preferred solving concrete problems." Anderson considered himself to be the "bacteria juggler" of the team while Smith

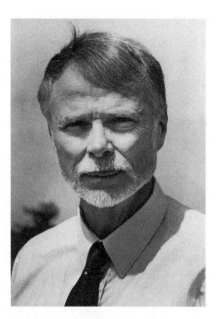

FIGURE 11.7 Porter Anderson, PhD.
Courtesy of the Albert and Mary Lasker Foundation.

"raised money and awareness."[61] As did many previous scientists, Smith and Anderson tested early versions of their vaccine on themselves and their colleagues before testing them on children.[62]

I recall Porter Anderson as intriguing, idiosyncratic, and very quiet. Although he didn't say much, when he spoke in his drawling Southern accent, it was worth stopping everything to listen. I agree with his colleague at Boston Children's, who found him "a brilliant, quirky fellow."[62] Anderson's attitude about his science reflects his unassuming ways:

> I am something of a night owl, and I tended to arrive late and stay late, working by myself. For the most part it was just doing one thing after another, putting things into test tubes and watching them change color. But there were moments of suspense and excitement, particularly in getting samples from people who had been vaccinated to see if they had a response or not.[62]

His words, in an understated way, capture the magic of scientific discovery.

The early *H. influenzae* vaccines, made of the purified polysaccharide antigen of Hib, did not generate strong, protective antibodies in young children.[52] Yet, very young children make high levels of long-lasting antibodies against protein antigens, such as tetanus and diphtheria toxoids. Smith and Anderson and Robbins and Schneerson wondered if they could trick babies' immature immune systems into generating immune responses to the capsule's sugar antigens as if they were proteins. Such a strategy might make better vaccines for young children.

The way to make a polysaccharide antigen act like a protein antigen was first recognized by Karl Landsteiner and James van der Scheer, who studied the roles of various chemical structures and configurations on their immunologic activities. The abilities of specific chemicals to stimulate a vigorous immune response depended on whether or not the chemicals were combined with a protein.[63] Subsequently, Oswald Avery and Walther Goebel applied Landsteiner and van der Scheer's principles to pneumococci by chemically combining the pneumococcal type III capsule with equine globulin, a protein isolated from the serum of a horse. Rabbits immunized with the type III capsule plus globulin antigen generated high levels of antibodies to the capsule, while those immunized with the capsule alone did not.[64] Thus, the inclusion of the globulin protein in the vaccine preparation changed the way the immune system of rabbits recognized and processed the polysaccharide capsule antigen.

This important experimental observation languished in laboratory file cabinets, however, for two reasons: (1) Adults generated antibodies to pneumococcal capsules without difficulty and (2) young children's inability to mount long-lasting antibodies against capsules was largely ignored. Babies, however, continued to die or suffer severe neurologic damage from *H. influenzae* meningitis. Motivated by those ill children, Schneerson and colleagues, building on Avery and Goebel's work, conjugated (i.e., chemically combined) the capsule of *H. influenzae* to several proteins, including albumin, hemocyanin, and diphtheria toxin. Schneerson observed that binding protein to the Hib capsule improved antibody responses to the capsule in immunized mice and rabbits.[65]

Three years later, Porter Anderson showed the same results in rabbits immunized with Hib capsule bound to a different protein by a different conjugation technique. He chose the nontoxic, mutant diphtheria toxin CRM197 as the conjugating protein because infants readily make antibodies to diphtheria toxoid vaccines.[66] In subsequent experiments, Anderson's preparation generated good antibody responses in young children as well.[67] Thus, both the Robbins/Schneerson and the Smith/Anderson teams worked feverishly to produce vaccines of Hib capsules conjugated to different proteins.

It was a race to the finish, and in the end Smith and Anderson beat Robbins and Schneerson. The CRM197-based Hib conjugate vaccine of Smith and Anderson was the first one shown to generate strong anti-PRP antibodies in infants. It was licensed in the United States in 1987. Schneerson and Robbins's vaccine, in which the Hib capsule was conjugated to tetanus toxoid, was licensed 6 years later. The work of these four scientists in developing conjugated Hib vaccines to protect babies against Hib meningitis had a tremendous impact on children's health. For their important discoveries, in 1996 all four scientists, Smith, Anderson, Robbins, and Schneerson, were awarded the prestigious Albert Lasker Clinical Medical Research Award.[68]

The success of the conjugate Hib vaccines has been spectacular. Prior to their introduction, an estimated 10,000 cases of Hib meningitis occurred annually in the United States,[69] which was approximately 1 in 300 children. It was even higher among native Alaskan and Native American Indian children.[70–72] Since the widespread use of the vaccine, the disease has nearly disappeared in the United States, with only 40 cases in children under age 5 years reported by the Centers for Disease Control and Prevention in 2014 (Figure 11.8).[73] This is likely a low estimate, however, as 266 cases in that same age group did not have the serotype of the *H. influenzae* reported, and at least some of them were probably type b.

Unfortunately, not all young American children are fully immunized, and those unimmunized remain at risk of serious infection with Hib. In 2014, three unvaccinated children from Missouri—two were 13 months old and the other 2 years old—developed serious *H. influenzae* infections (one had meningitis), and one died.[74]

The miracle of conjugating bacterial capsules to proteins didn't stop at *H. influenzae*. Using similar technology to conjugate sugars to proteins, vaccines to protect infants from meningitis caused by 13 serotypes

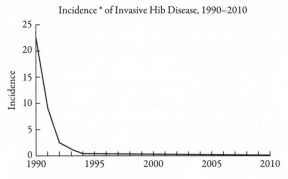

FIGURE 11.8 Incidence of *Haemophilus influenzae* type b (Hib) disease in the United States with the introduction of the conjugated Hib vaccines (1987).

From Centers for Disease Control and Prevention. The Pink Book: *Haemophilus influenzae* type b. 2015. https://www.cdc.gov/vaccines/pubs/pinkbook/hib.html.

of pneumococci[75] and 4 serogroups of meningococci[76] have subsequently been developed and are widely used in the United States and other developed countries. Thus, bacterial meningitis, once a scourge that killed and damaged too many American children, is, for the most part, now a bad memory.

References

1. Silhavy TJ, Kahne D, Walker S. The Bacterial Cell Envelope. *Cold Spring Harbor Perspectives in Biology.* 2010;2(5):a000414.
2. Frankland P. *Pasteur.* London: Cassell; 1901.
3. Pasteur L. Méthode pour Prévenir la Rage après Morsure. *Comptes Rendus des Séances de l'Académie des Sciences.* 1885;101:765–772.
4. Vallery-Radot R. *The Life of Pasteur.* New York: McClure Phillips; 1906.
5. Enders JF, Weller TH, Robbins FC. Cultivation of the Lansing Strain of Poliomyelitis Virus in Cultures of Various Human Embryonic Tissues. *Science.* 1949;109(2822):85–87.
6. Plotkin S. History of Vaccination. *Proceedings of the National Academy of Sciences of the United States of America.* 2014;111(34):12283–12287.
7. Enders JF, Katz SL, Milovanovic MV, Holloway A. Studies on an Attenuated Measles-Virus Vaccine. *New England Journal of Medicine.* 1960;263(4):153–159.

8. Centers for Disease Control and Prevention. Mumps. *The Pink Book*. 2015. https://www.cdc.gov/vaccines/pubs/pinkbook/mumps.html. Accessed March 2, 2017.

9. Plotkin SA, Farquhar JD, Katz M, Buser F. Attenuation of RA 27/3 Rubella Virus in WI-38 Human Diploid Cells. *American Journal of Diseases of Children*. 1969;118(2):178–185.

10. Takahashi M, Okuno Y, Otsuka T, Osame J, Takamizawa A. Development of a Live Attenuated Varicella Vaccine. *Biken Journal*. 1975;18(1):25–33.

11. Centers for Disease Control and Prevention. Measles. *The Pink Book*. 2015. https://www.cdc.gov/vaccines/pubs/pinkbook/meas.html. Accessed March 2, 2017.

12. Centers for Disease Control and Prevention. Hepatitis A. *The Pink Book*. 2015. https://www.cdc.gov/vaccines/pubs/pinkbook/hepa.html. Accessed March 2, 2017.

13. Provost PJ, Hughes JV, Miller WJ, Giesa PA, Banker FS, Emini EA. An Inactivated Hepatitis A Viral Vaccine of Cell Culture Origin. *Journal of Medical Virology*. 1986;19(1):23–31.

14. Salk JE, Krech U, Youngner JS, Bennett BL, Lewis LJ, Bazeley PL. Formaldehyde Treatment and Safety Testing of Experimental Poliomyelitis Vaccines. *American Journal of Public Health and the Nations Health*. 1954;44(5):563–570.

15. Centers for Disease Control and Prevention. Poliomyelitis. *The Pink Book*. 2015. https://www.cdc.gov/vaccines/pubs/pinkbook/polio.html. Accessed March 2, 2017.

16. Francis T, Napier JA, Voight RB, National Foundation for Infantile Paralysis. *Evaluation of the 1954 Field Trial of Poliomyelitis Vaccine: Final Report*. Ann Arbor, MI: Edward Brothers; 1957.

17. Gilsdorf JR. Brad Missed the Miracle. *Journal of the American Medical Association*. 1995;274(6):443–443.

18. Sabin AB. Oral Poliovirus Vaccine: History of Its Development and Use and Current Challenge to Eliminate Poliomyelitis from the World. *The Journal of Infectious Diseases*. 1985;151(3):420–436.

19. Blumberg BS, Friedlaender JS, Woodside A, Sutnick AI, London WT. Hepatitis and Australia Antigen: Autosomal Recessive Inheritance of Susceptibility to Infection in Humans. *Proceedings of the National Academy of Sciences of the United States of America*. 1969;62(4):1108–1115.

20. Blumberg BS. Australia Antigen and the Biology of Hepatitis B. *Science*. 1977;197(4298):17–25.

21. Hilleman MR, McAleer WJ, Buynak EB, McLean AA. The Preparation and Safety of Hepatitis B Vaccine. *Journal of Infection*. 1983;7:3–8.

22. Valenzuela P, Medina A, Rutter WJ, Ammerer G, Hall BD. Synthesis and Assembly of Hepatitis B Virus Surface Antigen Particles in Yeast. *Nature*. 1982;298(5872):347–350.

23. Centers for Disease Control and Prevention. Hepatitis B. *The Pink Book.* 2015. https://www.cdc.gov/vaccines/pubs/pinkbook/hepb.html. Accessed March 2, 2017.

24. Kirnbauer R, Booy F, Cheng N, Lowy DR, Schiller JT. Papillomavirus L1 Major Capsid Protein Self-Assembles into Virus-Like Particles that Are Highly Immunogenic. *Proceedings of the National Academy of Sciences of the United States of America.* 1992;89(24):12180–12184.

25. Lasker Foundation. HPV Vaccines for Cancer Prevention. 2017. http://www.laskerfoundation.org/awards/show/hpv-vaccines-cancer-prevention/. Accessed April 15, 2019.

26. von Behring E, Kitasato S. Uber das Zustandekommen Der Diphtherie-Immunitat Und der Tetanus-Immunitat Bei Thieren. In: Brock TD, ed., trans. *Milestones in Microbiology: 1556 to 1940.* Washington, DC: ASM Press; 1890:138.

27. Glenny AT, Hopkins BE. Diphtheria Toxoid as an Immunising Agent. *British Journal of Experimental Pathology.* 1923;4(5):283–288.

28. Descombey P. Tetanus Anatoxin. *Comptes Rendus des Seances de la Societe de Biologie.* 1924;91:239–241.

29. Madsen T. Vaccination Against Whooping Cough. *Journal of the American Medical Association.* 1933;101(3):187–188.

30. Sato Y, Sato H. Development of Acellular Pertussis Vaccines. *Biologicals.* 1999;27(2):61–69.

31. Centers for Disease Control and Prevention. Pertussis. *The Pink Book.* 2015. https://www.cdc.gov/vaccines/pubs/pinkbook/pert.html. Accessed March 2 2017.

32. Wright A, Parry Morgan W, Colebrook L, Dodgson RW. Observations on Prophylactic Inoculation Against Pneumococcus Infections, and on the Results Which Have Been Achieved by It. *The Lancet.* 1914; 183(4714):1–10.

33. Grabenstein JD, Klugman KP. A Century of Pneumococcal Vaccination Research in Humans. *Clinical Microbiology and Infection.* 2012;18: 15–24.

34. Tillett WS, Francis T. Serological Reactions in Pneumonia with a Non-Protein Somatic Fraction of Pneumococcus. *The Journal of Experimental Medicine.* 1930;52(4):561–571.

35. Felton LD. Studies on Immunizing Substances in Pneumococci VII. Response in Human Beings to Antigenic Pneumococcus Polysaccharides, Types I and II. *Public Health Reports.* 1938;53(42):1855–1905.

36. MacLeod CM, Hodges RG, Heidelberger M, Bernhard WG. Prevention of Pneumococcal Pneumonia by Immunization with Specific Capsular Polysaccharides. *The Journal of Experimental Medicine.* 1945;82(6):445–465.

37. Kaufman P. Pneumonia in Old Age: Active Immunization Against Pneumonia with Pneumococcus Polysaccharide; Results of a Six Year Study. *Archives of Internal Medicine.* 1947;79(5):518–531.

38. Butler JC, Shapiro ED, Carlone GM. Pneumococcal Vaccines: History, Current Status, and Future Directions. *The American Journal of Medicine.* 1999;107(1, Suppl. 1):69–76.

39. Watson DA, Daniel MM, Jacobson JW, Verhoef J. A Brief History of the Pneumococcus in Biomedical Research: A Panoply of Scientific Discovery. *Clinical Infectious Diseases.* 1993;17(5):913–924.

40. Geno KA, Gilbert GL, Song JY, et al. Pneumococcal Capsules and Their Types: Past, Present, and Future. *Clinical Microbiology Reviews.* 2015;28(3):871–899.

41. Gotschlich EC, Goldschneider I, Artenstein MS. Human Immunity to the Meningococcus. *Journal of Experimental Medicine.* 1969;129(6):1367–1384.

42. Goldschneider I, Gotschlich EC, Artenstein MS. Human Immunity to the Meningococcus. *Journal of Experimental Medicine.* 1969;129(6):1307–1326.

43. Centers for Disease Control and Prevention. Meningococcal Disease. *The Pink Book.* 2015. https://www.cdc.gov/vaccines/pubs/pinkbook/mening. html. Accessed March 2, 2017.

44. Stephens DS. Biology and Pathogenesis of the Evolutionarily Successful, Obligate Human Bacterium *Neisseria meningitidis.* *Vaccine.* 2009;27(Suppl. 2):B71–B77.

45. Zamenhof S, Leidy G, Fitzgerald PL, Alexander HE, Chargaff E. Polyribophosphate, the Type-Specific Substance of *Hemophilus influenzae*, Type b. *Journal of Biological Chemistry.* 1953;203(2):695–704.

46. Schneerson R, Rodrigues LP, Parke JC, Robbins JB. Immunity to Disease Caused by *Hemophilus influenzae* Type b: II Specificity and Some Biologic Characteristics of "Natural," Infection-Acquired, and Immunization-Induced Antibodies to the Capsular Polysaccharide of *Hemophilus influenzae* Type b. *Journal of Immunology.* 1971;107(4):1081–1089.

47. Anderson P, Peter G, Johnston RB, Wetterlow LH, Smith DH. Immunization of Humans with Polyribophosphate, the Capsular Antigen of *Hemophilus influenzae*, Type b. *Journal of Clinical Investigation.* 1972;51(1):39–44.

48. Centers for Disease Control and Prevention. *Haemophilus influenzae* type b. *The Pink Book.* 2015. https://www.cdc.gov/vaccines/pubs/pinkbook/hib. html. Accessed March 2, 2017.

49. Rodrigues LP, Schneerson R, Robbins JB. Immunity to *Hemophilus influenzae* Type b, I. The Isolation, and Some Physicochemical, Serologic and Biologic Properties of the Capsular Polysaccharide of *Hemophilus influenzae* Type b. *Journal of Immunology* 1971;107(4):1071–1080.

50. National Center for Biotechnology Information. Compound Summary Polyribosephosphate. PubChem CID 123744. 2005. https://pubchem.ncbi. nlm.nih.gov/compound/123744. Accessed March 25, 2017.

51. Fothergill LD, Wright J. Influenzal Meningitis: The Relation of Age Incidence to the Bacteridal Power of Blood against the Causal Organism. *Journal of Immunology.* 1933;24(4):273–284.

52. Smith DH, Peter G, Ingram DL, Harding AL, Anderson P. Responses of Children Immunized with the Capsular Polysaccharide of *Hemophilus influenzae*, Type b. *Pediatrics.* 1973;52(5):637–644.

53. Robbins JB, Parke JC, Schneerson R, Whisnant JK. Quantitative Measurement of Natural and Immunization-Induced *Haemophilus influenzas* type b Capsular Polysaccharide Antibodies. *Pediatric Research.* 1973;7(3):103–110.

54. Peltola H, Käythy H, Sivonen A, Mäkelä PH. *Haemophilus influenzae* Type b Capsular Polysaccharide Vaccine in Children: A Double-Blind Field Study of 100,000 Vaccinees 3 Months to 5 Years of Age in Finland. *Pediatrics.* 1977;60(5):730–737.

55. Robbins JB, Schneerson R, Porter A, Smith DH. Prevention of Systemic Infections, Especially Meningitis, Caused by *Haemophilus influenzae* Type b: Impact on Public Health and Implications for Other Polysaccharide-Based Vaccines. *Journal of the American Medical Association.* 1996;276(14):1181–1185.

56. Siber GR. Recognition of Excellence in Vaccinology and Global Immunization. Presentation of the Albert B. Sabin Gold Medal. 2001. http://www.sabin.org/sites/sabin.org/files/robbinsmedalspeech.pdf. Accessed March 24, 2017.

57. Rachel Schneerson. 2015. https://en.wikipedia.org/wiki/Rachel_Schneerson. Accessed March 24, 2017.

58. University of Rochester Medical Center. David H. Smith Center for Vaccine Biology and Immunology. About David H. Smith. 2017. https://www.urmc.rochester.edu/cvbi/history.aspx. Accessed March 18, 2017.

59. Freeman K. David H. Smith, 67, Developer of Vaccine Against Meningitis. *New York Times*, March 1, 1999. https://www.nytimes.com/1999/03/01/nyregion/david-h-smith-67-developer-of-vaccine-against-meningitis.html. Accessed July 26, 2019.

60. Society for Conservative Biology. David H. Smith: Visionary, Conservationist, Leader. 2017. http://conbio.org/mini-sites/smith-fellows/about-the-program/david-h.-smith. Accessed July 8, 2017.

61. Pearson D. The Problem Solver. *Emory Magazine*, Spring 2011. https://www.emory.edu/EMORY_MAGAZINE/issues/2011/spring/features/problem-solver/index.html. Accessed July 25, 2019.

62. Anderson T. Doctor on Team that Makes Hib Disease Rates Tumble: David Smith? http://www.scienceheroes.com/index.php?option=com_content&view=article&id=230&Itemid=230. Accessed March 18, 2017.

63. Landsteiner K, van der Scheer J. Serological Differentiation of Steric Isomers. *The Journal of Experimental Medicine.* 1928;48(3):315–320.

64. Avery OT, Goebel WF. Chemo-Immunological Studies on Conjugated Carbohydrate-Proteins. *Journal of Experimental Medicine* 1931;54(3):437–447.

65. Schneerson R, Barrera O, Sutton A, Robbins JB. Preparation, Characterization, and Immunogenicity of *Haemophilus influenzae* Type b

Polysaccharide-Protein Conjugates. *The Journal of Experimental Medicine.* 1980;152(2):361–376.

66. Anderson P. Antibody Responses to *Haemophilus influenzae* Type b and Diphtheria Toxin Induced by Conjugates of Oligosaccharides of the Type b Capsule with the Nontoxic Protein CRM197. *Infection and Immunity.* 1983;39(1):233–238.

67. Anderson P, Pichichero ME, Insel RA. Immunogens Consisting of Oligosaccharides from the Capsule of *Haemophilus influenzae* Type b Coupled to Diphtheria Toxoid or the Toxin Protein CRM197. *Journal of Clinical Investigation.* 1985;76(1):52–59.

68. Lasker Foundation. Vaccine for Preventing Meningitis in Children. 1996. http://www.laskerfoundation.org/awards/show/vaccine-for-preventing-meningitis-in-children/. Accessed March 22, 1917.

69. Parke JC Jr, Schneerson R, Robbins JB. The Attack Rate, Age Incidence, Racial Distribution, and Case Fatality Rate of *Hemophilus influenzae* Type b Meningitis in Mecklenburg County, North Carolina. *The Journal of Pediatrics.* 1972;81(4):765–769.

70. Gilsdorf JR. Bacterial Meningitis in Southwestern Alaska. *American Journal of Epidemiology.* 1977;106(5):388–391.

71. Losonsky GA, Santosham M, Sehgal VM, Zwahlen A, Moxon ER. *Haemophilus influenzae* Disease in the White Mountain Apaches: Molecular Epidemiology of a High Risk Population. *Pediatric Infectious Diseases Journal.* 1984;3(6):539–547.

72. Coulehan JL, Michaels RH, Hallowell C, Schults R, Welty TK, Kuo JS. Epidemiology of *Haemophilus influenzae* Type B Disease Among Navajo Indians. *Public Health Reports (Washington, DC: 1974).* 1984;99(4):404–409.

73. Adams DA, Thomas KR, Jajosky RA, et al. Summary of Notifiable Infectious Diseases and Conditions—United States, 2014. *MMWR Morbidity and Mortality Weekly Report.* 2016;63:1–152.

74. Myers AL, Jackson MA, Zhang L, Swanson DS, Gilsdorf JR. *Haemophilus influenzae* Type b Invasive Disease in Amish Children, Missouri, USA, 2014. *Emerging Infectious Diseases.* 2017;23(1):112–114.

75. Black S, Shinefield H, Fireman B, et al. Efficacy, Safety and Immunogenicity of Heptavalent Pneumococcal Conjugate Vaccine in Children. *The Pediatric Infectious Disease Journal.* 2000;19(3):187–195.

76. Bilukha OO, Rosenstein N. Prevention and Control of Meningococcal Disease. *MMWR Recommendations and Reports.* 2005;54(RR07):1–21.

12

A Scientist and a Scientist Walk into a Bar

BY THE MID-1990S, *Haemophilus influenzae* meningitis was rare in the United States. The *H. influenzae* type b (Hib) vaccine—that magical sugar from the capsule conjugated to a protein—worked exceptionally well to protect babies against *H. influenzae* meningitis, and parents across America eagerly immunized their infants. No longer were thousands of children damaged from this disease every year. Scientific work on *H. influenzae* and the other bacteria that cause meningitis in young children continued, however, as many important questions remain about how they, and other microbes, cause meningitis. The answers to many of these questions rest in the genes buried deep in the chromosomes of the bacteria.

In the spring of 1993, Hamilton Smith, the Nobel Prize–winning scientist who discovered site-specific, DNA-cutting restriction enzymes in *H. influenzae*, chaired a session at a meeting in Bilbao, Spain, that had been convened to discuss various scientific, legal, and religious aspects of the still-infantile Human Genome Project, the massive project to identify all human genes. At the end of one of the meeting days, Smith headed to the hotel's bar for a drink. There he ran into Dr. Craig Venter, who had spoken at one of the earlier sessions. They began to talk science. Venter had just started an institute focused on genomic medicine, and in his previous position at the National Institutes of Health (NIH), he had developed an automated method to sequence DNA. Venter's new method, called expressed sequence tags (ESTs), identified the complete nucleotide sequences of genes related to brain function

Continual Raving: A History of Meningitis and the People Who Conquered It. Janet R Gilsdorf, Oxford University Press (2020). © Oxford University Press.
DOI: 10.1093/oso/9780190677312.001.0001

more quickly than the established methods.[1] Smith and Venter talked and talked far into the night.[2]

Craig Venter (Figure 12.1) was born in Salt Lake City, Utah, and grew up in Millbrae, California, a small city wedged between the San Francisco airport and the San Andreas reservoir, which sits directly atop the famous fault. A risk-taker from early childhood, young Craig, aboard his bicycle, used to chase airplanes as they took off from the airport.[3] School wasn't his favorite activity, and he was such a poor student that his worried mother sometimes checked his arms for needle tracks.[4] After graduating from high school, he joined the navy and served as a medical corpsman in Vietnam. This proved to be a formative experience that drove his subsequent interest in medicine and biology.

Following his military service, he attended community college and then the University of California San Diego as a premed major. Somewhere along the line, his interest in medical school faded, and he ended up with a bachelor's degree in chemistry, followed by a PhD in physiology and pharmacology.[5] After 8 years on the faculty at the State

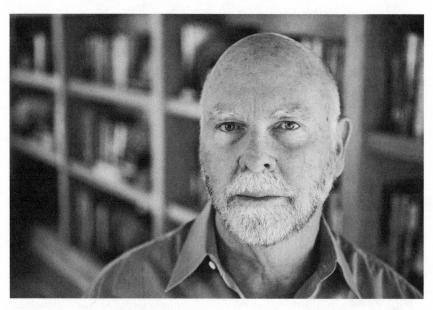

FIGURE 12.1 Dr. Craig Venter.
Courtesy of the J. Craig Venter Institute.

University of New York at Buffalo, Venter became chief of the Section of Receptor Biochemistry and Molecular Biology at the National Institute of Neurological Disorders and Stroke at the NIH. There, his research focused on genes that encode enzymes involved in the synthesis of neurotransmitters and their receptors in the brain.

In 1992, Venter left the NIH, possibly related to a dust-up involving the US Patent and Trademark Office (USPTO). He and the NIH had tried to patent his EST technique, and the USPTO rejected the application, stating that the invention wasn't novel, and the claims were vague and indefinitive.[6] Further, after several legal appeals, the NIH withdrew the application because such patents were "not in the best interests of the public or science."[7] When Venter encountered Ham Smith in the Spanish bar, he had just started The Institute for Genomic Research (TIGR), the first of a number of his genomic business ventures.

At the invitation of Venter, Smith visited TIGR in Gaithersburg, Maryland, and was "blown away" by Venter's operation.[2] Thirty DNA sequencers, each the size of a washing machine, housed in a gigantic, 26,000-square-foot room, were cranking out DNA sequences at the rate of 400,000 base pairs a day, considerably faster than conventional sequencing techniques. When he realized the potential of Venter's system, Smith suggested Venter conduct a proof-of-principle experiment to demonstrate the feasibility of ESTs for generating gene sequences by testing the genome a freely living organism. Smith told Venter he should focus on the chromosomal DNA of a bacterium. "We can sequence it in only 2 weeks," he told Venter and recommended they use *H. influenzae* because of its relatively small size, because the ratio of guanidine plus cytidine-containing nucleotides is similar to that of humans, and because a physical clone map of the bacteria didn't exist.[8]

To get started on the sequencing project, Smith handed Venter a vial of *H. influenzae* strain Rd, the strain Hattie Alexander had used in her DNA transformation experiments, and Venter went to work. His hypothesis was that segments of DNA as large as a bacterial chromosome could be sequenced rapidly, accurately, and cost effectively. In 2 years, the project was complete, and the paper was published in *Science* magazine, with a color-coded map of the entire gene structure of the bacterium printed on the cover (Figure 12.2).[8] The paper not only detailed each gene in *H. influenzae* strain Rd but also catalogued the likely function of each

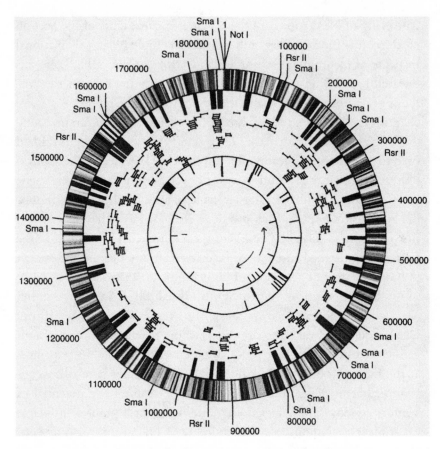

FIGURE 12.2 Cartoon of all the genes in the *H. influenzae* strain Rd chromosome.

From Fleishmann RD, Adams MD, White O, et al. Whole-Genome Random Sequencing and Assembly of *Haemophilus influenzae* Rd. *Science*. 1995;269:496–512. Courtesy of *Science*.

gene. This was the first complete DNA sequence of a free-living organism to be characterized, and it opened up a world of new opportunities for scientists who studied these, and similar, bacteria. With the genome map in hand, they could mutate specific genes and test the impact of the mutations on bacterial metabolism, physiology, and pathogenicity.

After the completion of the *H. influenzae* genome sequence, Venter turned TIGR over to Dr. Claire Fraser, a noted molecular biologist and, at that time, his wife, and founded Celera Genomics, a company devoted to sequencing the human genome. This project was in direct competition with one led by Dr. Francis Collins from the NIH, whose scientists and many international collaborators were also sequencing the human genome. The rivalry was ferocious. Venter's new way of sequencing was much faster than the clunky older method of Collins and his collaborators. The human genome sequence was declared complete in 2003, with Collins and Venter given equal credit for its completion (Figure 12.3). Collins and his international collaborators published their sequence in the journal *Nature* on February 15, 2001,[9] and Venter published his in the journal *Science* on February 16, 2001.[10]

Following completion of that monumental project, the board of Celera fired Venter in the midst of disputes about its profitability.[4] Subsequently, Venter combined several of his businesses and founded the J. Craig Venter Institute (JCVI) with multiple goals that included sequencing organisms from ocean samples, from the human microbiome (all bacteria living in and on humans), and from a number of infectious disease transmission vectors, such as mosquitoes. In addition, they began working on creating the first synthetic chromosome.[11]

To say that Venter is a complicated person is an understatement. In addition to his work as a gene jockey, he is an author. In 2007, his autobiography, *A Life Decoded: My Genome—My Life,* was published. The title is a double entendre, referring both to his work in decoding genomes and to the fact that the human genome sequenced by his company TIGR contained DNA from five individuals, including himself. The ethicist Arthur Caplan, in reviewing the book, described it as "400 pages of egocentric prose." Yet, Caplan, accurately, considers Venter to be "a friend, a brilliant scientist, an extraordinary entrepreneur, and a true visionary when it comes to genomics."[3]

Since Richard Pfeiffer first spotted his influenza bacilli in the respiratory secretions of patients suffering from influenza during the Russian pandemic, scientists of all stripes have built, one discovery at a time, a monument to understanding how *H. influenzae* as well as pneumococci and meningococci cause bacterial meningitis. The culmination of these many, diverse efforts is the near disappearance of this dreadful infection, at least in countries that provide vaccines to their young citizens. Earlier, smallpox, diphtheria, tetanus, whooping cough, measles,

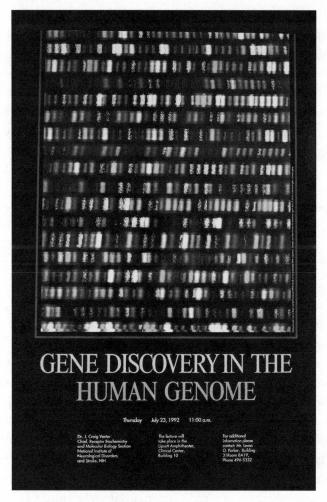

FIGURE 12.3 Poster announcing Dr. Craig Venter's lecture on gene discovery in the human genome, 1992.

From the NIH US National Library of Medicine. Gene Discovery in the Human Genome. https://collections.nlm.nih.gov/catalog/nlm:nlmuid-101454172-img.

and polio became almost nonexistent in America because of a tower of scientific knowledge and the use of vaccines that emerged from that knowledge. Now, meningitis is almost there. The continual raving of this infection has nearly been silenced.

More discoveries lay ahead—many more. Scientists continue to unearth the hidden mysteries of microbes, the myriad ways bacteria cope with the exigencies of their lives and how they discern strategies for winning the next battle, for finding the next meal, and for ensuring their perpetuity through the success of their offspring.

References

1. Adams MD, Kelley JM, Gocayne JD, et al. Complementary DNA Sequencing: Expressed Sequence Tags and Human Genome Project. *Science.* 1991;252(5013):1651–1656.
2. Gitschier J. A Half-Century of Inspiration: An Interview with Hamilton Smith. *PLoS Genetics.* 2012;8(1):e1002466.
3. Caplan AL. A Life Decoded: My Genome—My Life. *The Journal of Clinical Investigation.* 2008;118(3):828–828.
4. Herper M. Craig Venter Mapped the Genome. Now He's Trying to Decode Death. *Forbes.* 2017. https://www.forbes.com/sites/matthewherper/2017/02/21/can-craig-venter-cheat-death/#30c2740d1645. Accessed July 8, 2017.
5. Shampo MA, Kyle RA. J. Craig Venter—The Human Genome Project. *Mayo Clinic Proceedings.* 2011;86(4):e26–e27.
6. Kankanala KC. *Genetic Patent Law and Strategy.* Noida, India: Manupatra; 2007.
7. Anderson C. NIH Drops Bid for Gene Patents. *Science.* 1994;263(5149):909–910.
8. Fleischmann RD, Adams MD, White O, et al. Whole-Genome Random Sequencing and Assembly of *Haemophilus influenzae* Rd. *Science.* 1995;269(5223):496–512.
9. International Human Genome Sequencing Consortium. Initial Sequencing and Analysis of the Human Genome. *Nature.* 2001;409(6822):860–921.
10. Venter JC, Adams MD, Myers EW, et al. The Sequence of the Human Genome. *Science.* 2001;291(5507):1304–1351.
11. J. Craig Venter Institute. Research. 2019. https://www.jcvi.org/research. Accessed April 16, 2019.

Epilogue: Searching for Richard Pfeiffer

AS WE PLANNED A visit with our son Daniel, who lived, at that time, in Warsaw, I mentioned that Richard Pfeiffer, the man who discovered the bacteria I had studied my entire professional life, had retired and died in Poland. "He's buried in a place called Lądek Zdrój," I said. Instantly my son replied, "Mom, let's find his grave while you're here."

So, in April 2016, I, along with Dan and my husband, embarked on a quest to find Richard Pfeiffer's resting place. As we rode the express railway from Warsaw to Wrocław (previously known as Breslau), we passed the backyards and junkyards of rural Poland along the way. The clotheslines, the gardens, and the leftovers of bygone days zipped past the train windows. The land was flat and fertile, the fields neatly tilled, the homes well maintained.

In Wrocław, we rented a car for the drive to Bad Landeck, where Dr. Fildes (1956), in his memorial to Dr. Pfeiffer, said Pfeiffer was buried. The village, founded around 1280 and now called Lądek Zdrój, is located in Lower Silesia near the Czech border and has a population of approximately 6,000 people. The region has long been a popular resort area because of its mineral springs and health spas. As we approached the town, the fields gave way to the hazy foothills of the Sudentan Mountains, dotted with stands of evergreens and budding trees.

A Polish friend of our son had recommended we stay at the Proharmonia Residence, a lovely mansion turned inn nestled into the thicket at the edge of town. From the window in our room, I stared at the aspens, fir, pine, and beech trees that stretched up the hill. Squirrels scurried from branch to branch. The woods, deep and mysterious, reminded me of fairy-tale forests, of Hansel and Gretel, of Goldilocks and the Three Bears, of Little Red Riding Hood and the Wolf.

Continual Raving: A History of Meningitis and the People Who Conquered It. Janet R Gilsdorf, Oxford University Press (2020). © Oxford University Press.
DOI: 10.1093/oso/9780190677312.001.0001

The receptionists at Proharmonia knew nothing of Dr. Richard Pfeiffer, but they gave us a town map that showed two crosses beside the village church indicating a cemetery. Fildes had said Pfeiffer was buried in the "parish cemetery," so it seemed a good start for our search. When we arrived at the Church of the Nativity of the Blessed Virgin Mary, however, we found only a few, very old gravestones embedded into the wall of the surrounding garden, and none belonged to Richard Pfeiffer. We headed to the town cemetery, a few blocks from the church, and learned that it is actually two cemeteries, the parish cemetery containing graves of Roman Catholic church members and the community cemetery with graves of the others. At the far end of the Catholic cemetery stood a small chapel (Figure E1).

As we walked between the crowded rows of tombs and wondered how we would ever find Pfeiffer among all those graves, we noted they were new, most since 2000. All were generously decorated with plastic flowers and candles in glass jars, and some had wooden benches. A groundskeeper was picking up broken glass and crumbled flowers, and Dan asked, in his rudimentary Polish, about graves from 1945, the year of Pfeiffer's death. She told him, in very broken English—we hoped we understood her correctly—that old graves are replaced by new ones after about 20 years. At one end of the community graveyard, we found a few older tombstones stacked against the fence, many broken and etched with illegible engravings—no Richard Pfeiffer.

Empty handed, we left the cemetery and strolled through the village center. As we passed the town hall, I spotted a sign with a green arrow that said, "Biblioteka" (library) and figured the town librarian might know something about Pfeiffer. The lady at the desk in the lending room—it was a very small library—referred us to the lady in the information room, whose scowl intensified as she increasingly understood our question and then leafed through a large book on her desk. Finally, she made a phone call, chatted in rapid-fire Polish for a short minute, and then explained that someone would call us by 5 that afternoon if they found anything.

The call came the next morning; the librarians uncovered no public records about Richard Pfeiffer. The language barrier, however, prohibited knowing exactly what that meant. Discouraged by our failure to find his grave, we spent about an hour drinking beer (the men)/Pepsi

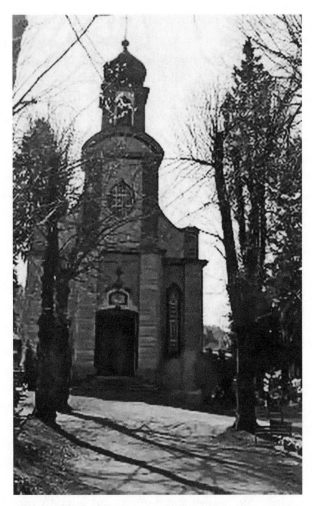

FIGURE E1 Chapel in the cemetery where Richard Pfeiffer was buried.
Photograph by the author.

(me) at a tiny local bar on the town square. Then, we stopped for lunch
in a Polish pizza place, curiously called Abakus, one of the few eating es-
tablishments in downtown Lądek Zdrój. They had run out of pierogis,
so we ordered a pizza with kielbasa, onions, and dill pickles. Neither the
guy at the counter nor the waitress spoke English, but a fellow named
Marcin, a friend of the owner, leaned on the bar and explained, in excellent English, that he grew up in Lądek Zdrój, had lived in Madrid
for 20 years, and was back in town for his grandmother's funeral. He

seemed eager to speak with Americans and offered to help in the search for the grave. He suggested we return to the church.

Marcin, whose mother worked for the parish priest, met us at the Church of the Nativity of the Blessed Virgin Mary and explained our mission to the official who answered the door. The rector eventually warmed to us. He disappeared into a closet stuffed with, among other things, boxes of candles, a bicycle, a vacuum cleaner, a fan, a mop and bucket, a film projector, and a portable screen and returned with a massive ledger of deaths among parishioners since 1900. Each death had been carefully recorded (name, date, and other information we couldn't read) in neat, black-ink script—no Richard Pfeiffer in all of 1945. As we were about to leave, he invited us into the closet and pulled out several much older ledgers. Turns out that all of the death ledgers since the establishment of the church, in the 1300s, stood, not in a safe or a fireproof vault, but there on dusty shelves in the back of that closet.

The next stop in our search for Pfeiffer was 5 Konopnickiej Street, reported by Cieślik[1] and an anonymous contributor to Wikipedia[2] to be the location of his home, which he called "Heimatsonne," loosely translated as sunny home. We found that the address plate on the side of the house that sits between the one marked number 6 and the Villa Rosa marked number 4 had been replaced with a blank tile. The presumptive 5 Konopnickiej looked identical to the pale salmon stucco home with a red-tiled roof pictured in the Wikipedia photos. Beside the house was the garden, edged by a hedge, that Fildes mentioned in his memorial to Pfeiffer.[3] Four garbage cans stood at the clean, tidy curb.

It was a warm, sunny spring afternoon, and several windows of the house were open; their dainty lace curtains fluttered like dove wings in the breeze. In the days when Pfeiffer lived there, we would have heard his piano music—likely he would have played Chopin—wafting from behind those curtains. There, on the other side of the second floor windows, was where Pfeiffer was forced to live when the Polish troops occupied his home (Figure E2).

Standing on the sidewalk outside the house, I imagined the elderly Pfeiffer, aided by a cane and his housekeeper, Frau Köhler, slowly shuffling up to Stanislaw Moniuszko Park about four blocks away (Figure E3). He might have climbed the park's hill to the Chapel of St. Jerzy with its octagonal, freestanding bell tower. He probably

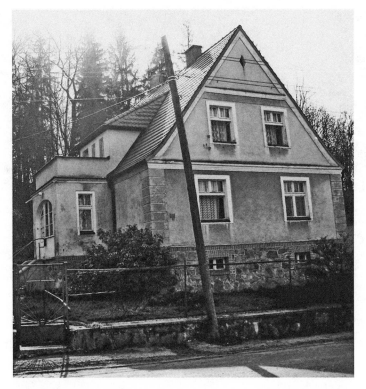

FIGURE E2 Richard Pfeiffer's retirement home in Lądek Zdrój.
Photograph by the author.

wandered beside the banks of the rocky Biała Lądecka River that bur-
bles through town and crossed over the ancient St. John's Bridge. He
likely listened to the cooing of the wood pigeons and the tolling of
the church bells and the rustle of the aspen leaves. He would have had
a peaceful, serene life in this peaceful, serene village after his highly
productive life as professor in the much larger, much busier, city of
Wrocław.

As I snapped several pictures of Pfeiffer's house, I heard the voices of
women beyond the garden. They sounded neither young nor friendly.
Likely they were suspicious of a stranger walking up and down the
sidewalk, taking photos. The Poles have suffered mightily under repres-
sive governments, over and over, and older women, like those, would
understandably be wary. When I rejoined my son, he said, "Mom,
those ladies were giving you the serious stink eye."

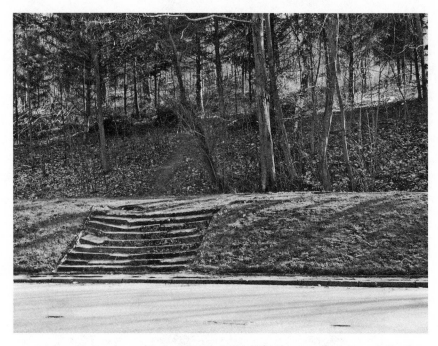

FIGURE E3 Steps along the path Richard Pfeiffer would have walked to enter the park in Lądek Zdrój.
Photograph by the author.

In the end, we found Richard Pfeiffer's house, but not his grave. I suspect his death wasn't recorded in the Catholic Church ledger because he was the son of a Protestant minister and likely wasn't a member of the Roman Catholic parish. If he attended church at all, he may have been a member of the Evangelical Church of the Savior in Lądek Zdrój, which was abandoned after World War II when most of the Protestant Germans fled the town[4]. In 1999, the church burned and is now an eerie, roofless, hollow shell (Figure E4). There were no graves in the tiny yard that surrounds its charred stone skeleton.

After returning to the United States, I found photos of Pfeiffer's house on WikiMedia that had been posted by Maciej Miezian, an art historian at the Historical Museum in Krakow.[5] I sent him a message through Facebook, asking about Richard Pfeiffer's grave. He quickly responded and, apologizing for his limited English, explained that his wife is from Lądek Zdrój. He said that Pfeiffer was buried in what

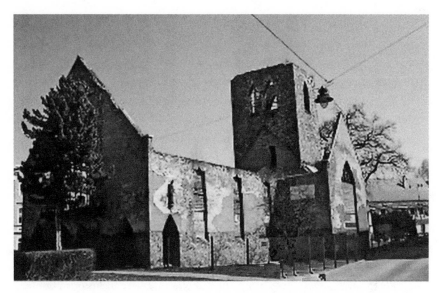

FIGURE E4   Remains of the Evangelical Church of the Savior in Lądek Zdrój.
Photograph by the author.

is now the Catholic parish cemetery but was previously a Protestant cemetery, and that the grave was destroyed in 1960. He confirmed that it was plowed under by the Soviets following World War II.[6]

With a little research, I learned the complexities of burials in Lądek Zdrój. The first cemetery was built in 1616 because the graveyard surrounding the Catholic church, originally built in the thirteenth century, was overcrowded. In the 1880s, the parish cemetery was expanded to include acreage a short distance to the south. Thirty years later, an Evangelical cemetery and chapel were built to the south of the expansion, and a small Jewish cemetery was established just south of the Evangelical cemetery and remained open until 1933. In 1945, the Communists took over the original Catholic cemetery and used it as a nonsectarian municipal cemetery, as it remains today. In 1970, what had been the Evangelical cemetery and chapel merged with the expanded Catholic cemetery into today's Catholic parish cemetery and chapel. All that remains of the Jewish cemetery are short sections of a stone fence. Oddly, since 1993, the graves are reused 20 years after a burial.[7]

Although Richard Pfeiffer was no longer there, we had tumbled on Marcin and found clues to Pfeiffer's final days. We strolled the grounds of the quiet place where Pfeiffer was laid to rest in the chaotic time at the end of World War II. In the sweet sunlight of Lądek Zdrój, we had breathed the air of his beloved little village and stood beside the knee-high stone wall that surrounded his house. His days at Heimatsonne had been a peaceful ending to Richard Pfeiffer's productive life, a chance for him to reflect on his important additions to the understanding of microbes, on the miracle of living things, on the beauty of scientific inquiry. He, as much as anyone, had known the rewards of discovery.

References

1. Cieślik G. Historia Lądka Zdroju w latach w XIX w. *Lądek Zdrój– Nieoficjalna strona.* 2000. http://ladekzdroj.w.interiowo.pl/historia4.html. Accessed July 2017.
2. Richard Friedrich Johannes Pfeiffer. 2006. https://en.wikipedia.org/wiki/ Richard_Friedrich_Johannes_Pfeiffer. Accessed July 13, 2017.
3. Fildes P. Richard Friedrich Johannes Pfeiffer. 1858–1945. *Biographical Memoirs of Fellows of the Royal Society.* 1956;2:237–247.
4. Parish Cemetery in Lądek Zdrój. https://translate.googleusercontent. com/translate_c?depth=1&hl=en&prev=search&rurl=translate.google. com&sl=pl&u=https://pl.m.wikipedia.org/wiki/Cmentarz_parafialny_w_ L%25C4%2585dku-Zdroju&usg=ALkJrhhd7CnCuFnLfceEE3Y3asTSPJ5 lVw. Accessed July 24, 2019.
5. Miezianas M. File: Lądek Zdrój, Richard Pfeiffer house.jpg. 2009. https:// commons.wikimedia.org/wiki/File:L%C4%85dek_Zdr%C3%B3j,_Richard_ Pfeiffer_house.jpg. Accessed July 8, 2017.
6. Ruczkowska J. What's Common About the Two Outstanding Researchers Richard Pfeiffer—Microbiologist and Albert Neisser—Dermatologist. *Advances in Clinical and Experimental Medicine.* 2005;14(3):635–636.
7. Iwona Dakiniewicz. Iwona's Sources-Cemeteries. 2010. http://www.ipgs.us/ iwonad/artdirectory/cemeteries.html. Accessed July 24, 2019. Accessed July 13, 2017.

GLOSSARY

—————⋙•◆•⋘—————

Adjuvant—An additive to vaccines that improves the immune response.

Agar—The jelly-like substance on which bacteria are propagated in the laboratory.

Agglutination—An immunological test that shows the clumping of bacteria when they are mixed with antisera directed toward antigens on those bacteria.

Anaphylaxis—A severe immune reaction to a foreign agent, such as a drug or serum, characterized by suffusion of the face, restlessness, increased heart rate, difficulty breathing, urticaria (hives), and, rarely, cardiovascular collapse.

Antibody—A protein in the blood that is produced by the immune system in response to an infection.

Antigen—A molecule on bacteria or viruses that stimulates an immune response, with resultant production of antibodies.

Antisera—The fraction of the blood in immunized subjects that contains antibodies against the immunizing agent.

Attenuated—Altered by heating or chemical treatments or genetic manipulation.

Bactericidal—Destructive to bacteria.

Bacteriophage—A virus that infects bacteria.

Biotype—The shared genetic composition of clusters of biologic subspecies that have similar characteristics.

Capsule—The sugar-containing structure that surrounds strains of *Haemophilus influenzae*, pneumococci, and meningococci that cause meningitis.

Carbohydrate—Another name for a sugar.

Cellulitis—Infection of the skin and underlying soft tissues.

Colonies of bacteria—Mounds of bacteria growing on agar plates.

Complement—A protein in the blood that enhances the ability of antibodies to kill bacteria.

CSF—Cerebrospinal fluid; clear liquid that surrounds the brain and spinal cord.

Culture—The process of growing bacteria in the laboratory from clinical specimens.

Empiric antibiotics——Antimicrobial treatment given to a patient with an infection before the cause of the infection has been identified.

Encapsulated—Bacteria possessing a capsule made of complex sugars.

Endocarditis—Infection of one of the valves of the heart.

Enzymes—Biologically active proteins.

Epiglottitis—Inflammation of the epiglottis, the flap of tissue that covers the bronchus when swallowing to prevent food from descending into the lungs.

Etiology—Cause.

Fulminant infection—An infection that rapidly progresses in severity, sometimes culminating in death.

Hib—*Haemophilus influenzae* type b.

Horizontal gene transfer—The process of passing genetic material from one bacterium to another.

Meninges—The three membranes (dura mater, pia mater, and arachnoid mater) that surround the brain and spinal column.

Meningitis—Infection of the meninges.

Miasmic—Refers to the theory that attributed the cause of disease to bad air.

Morphoforms—The different physical shapes assumed by colonies of the same bacterial species.

Necrotizing cellulitis—Infection of the skin that results in death of the tissue.

Neurovirulence—Toxicity for nervous tissues.

Neutrophil—A type of white blood cell that ingests and digests foreign biologic material, including bacteria.

Nonencapsulated—Bacteria with no capsule.

Nucleotides—The five subunits of DNA or RNA: adenine, thymine, guanine, cytosine, and uracil.

Opsonization—The ability of immune serum factors to promote phagocytosis of bacteria by neutrophils.

Osteomyelitis—Infection of a bone.

Otitis media—Infection of the middle ear, often called an "ear infection" in children.

Pathogenicity—The propensity of a bacterium to cause infection.

Phagocytic—The ability of a cell to ingest small foreign particles.

Phylogenetic—Refers to the evolutionary history and relationships of the biologic species under study.

Plasma—The colorless fluid of centrifuged blood that contains, among other proteins, antibodies and clotting factors.

Plasmid—Small, circular piece of DNA that travels from cell to cell in bacteria.

Pneumonia—Infection of the lung.

Polysaccharide—A large molecule composed of multiple sugar molecules.

Precipitation—An immunological test that shows fine precipitates when purified antigens are mixed with antisera directed against the antigen.

Restriction—The process that limits bacteria from taking up foreign DNA.

Restriction endonuclease—An enzyme that cuts apart DNA at specific nucleotides.

Septic arthritis—Infection of a joint.

Serum—The colorless fluid of clotted blood that contains, among other proteins, antibodies.

Sinusitis—Infection of one of the nasal sinuses.

Sputum (pleural sputa)—Secretion(s) from the lungs that are coughed up.

Subcutaneous—Beneath the skin.

Transformation—The ability of bacteria to take on new characteristics by acquiring new DNA.

Transposon—A small piece of DNA that hops from place to place in a chromosome; a "jumping gene."

Unencapsulated—Bacteria with no capsule.

Ventricles of the brain—Spaces deep in the brain that contain cerebrospinal fluid.

INDEX

Tables and figures are indicated by *t* and *f* following the page number

For the benefit of digital users, indexed terms that span two pages (e.g., 52–53) may, on occasion, appear on only one of those pages.